2 8 MAY 2022

Neuropsychology for Occupational Therapists

Assessment of Perception and Cognition

Second Edition

June Grieve
BSc, MSc

D0495330

YORK ST. JOHN
COLLEGE LIBRARY

Blackwell
Science

York St. John College

3 8025 00426659 2

© June Grieve 1993

Blackwell Science Ltd
Editorial Offices:
Osney Mead, Oxford OX2 0EL
25 John Street, London WC1N 2BS
23 Ainslie Place, Edinburgh EH3 6AJ
350 Main Street, Malden
   MA 02148 5018, USA
54 University Street, Carlton
   Victoria 3053, Australia

Other Editorial Offices:

Blackwell Wissenschafts-Verlag GmbH
Kurfürstendamm 57
10707 Berlin, Germany

Blackwell Science KK
MG Kodenmacho Building
7-10 Kodenmacho Nihombashi
Chuo-ku, Tokyo 104, Japan

Iowa State University Press
A Blackwell Science Company
2121 S. State Avenue
Ames, Iowa 50014-8300, USA

The right of the Author to be identified as
the Author of this Work has been asserted
in accordance with the Copyright, Designs
and Patents Act 1988.

All rights reserved. No part of this
publication may be reproduced, stored in
a retrieval system, or transmitted, in any
form or by any means, electronic,
mechanical, photocopying, recording or
otherwise, except as permitted by the UK
Copyright, Designs and Patents Act
1988, without the prior permission of the
publisher.

First published 1993
Reprinted 1995, 1996, 1997
Second edition 2000
Reprinted 2001

Set in 10/13 Times
by Aarontype Limited, Easton, Bristol
Printed and bound in Great Britain by MPG
Books Ltd, Bodmin, Cornwall

The Blackwell Science logo is a
trade mark of Blackwell Science Ltd,
registered at the United Kingdom
Trade Marks Registry

DISTRIBUTORS

Marston Book Services Ltd
PO Box 269
Abingdon Oxon OX14 4YN
(Orders: Tel: 01235 465500
        Fax: 01235 465555)
USA
Blackwell Science, Inc.
Commerce Place
350 Main Street
Malden, MA 02148 5018
(Orders: Tel: 800 759 6102
            781 388 8250
        Fax: 781 388 8255)
Canada
Login Brothers Book Company
324 Saulteaux Crescent
Winnipeg, Manitoba R3J 3T2
(Orders: Tel: 204 837 2987
        Fax: 204 837 3116)
Australia
Blackwell Science Pty Ltd
54 University Street
Carlton, Victoria 3053
(Orders: Tel: 03 9347-0300
        Fax: 03 9347-5001)

A catalogue record for this title
is available from the British Library
ISBN 0-632-05067-5

Library of Congress
Cataloging-in-Publication Data

Grieve, June I.
    Neuropsychology for occupational
  therapists: assessment of perception and
  cognition/June Grieve.—2nd ed.
  Includes bibliographical references and
  index.
  ISBN 0-632-05067-5 (pbk.)
    1. Neuropsychological tests. 2. Clinical
  neuropsychology. 3. Occupational therapy.
  4. Occupational therapists. I. Title.
  [DNLM: 1. Neuropsychology. 2. Cognition—
  physiology. 3. Cognition Disorders—
  diagnosis. 4. Memory Disorders—diagnosis.
  5. Motor Skills Disorders—diagnosis.
  6. Neurologic Examination. 7. Occupational
  Therapy. 8. Perception —physiology.
  WL 103 G848n 1999]
  RC386.6.N48 G75   1999
  616.8'0475—dc21

                                    99–051960

For further information on
Blackwell Science, visit our website:
www.blackwell-science.com

Contents

Foreword

Many changes have occurred in the profession since the first edition of this book. The introduction of primary care teams in the community has led to the creation of more specialist neurorehabilitation posts. For occupational therapists working in acute settings and in neurorehabilitation units there is continuing pressure to increase the throughput of beds which demands rigorous client assessment. At the same time, the move towards evidence-based practice requires the therapist to develop high-level assessment skills supported by appropriate standardized tests. In line with advances in technology, occupational therapists must be able to interpret the results of brain scans which can indicate prognosis and guide the planning of intervention.

The book provides the student with descriptions of perceptual and cognitive abilities, supported by theoretical models, in a clear and user-friendly style. Experienced clinicians will find more in-depth assessment of perceptual and cognitive deficits for their neurologically impaired clients, based on an understanding of the under-lying mechanisms. The effects of perceptual and cognitive impairment on function are considered, together with examples of relevant assessments which have been updated to include more standardized batteries of tests.

The clinician must never lose sight of the fact that the patient may present with multiple problems. No concrete answers are given. The reader is encouraged to use the information presented, and his/her clinical reasoning, to plan an appropriate assessment programme prior to intervention. Members of the multidisciplinary team will gain an insight into the unique role of the occupational therapist in the rehabilitation of cognitive deficits.

Jacqueline Adams
DipCOT, OTR

Preface

The aim of the first edition was to stimulate the interest of occupational therapy students and clinicians in the part played by cognition in daily living, and to encourage more assessment of cognitive problems in clients with neurological impairment. Over the six years since the first edition appeared, the developments in cognitive science within neuropsychology have included studies using imaging techniques which allow active brain areas to be identified during cognitive function. During this period, further standardized assessments of perception and cognition have also appeared, and more are currently under development.

This edition retains the format of the first. Part I serves as an introduction to the methods of cognitive neuropsychology and to the components of the complex cognitive system. Part II outlines the theoretical background to the individual cognitive abilities. The contents of this part are chosen selectively to reflect relevance to daily living, excluding behavioural, psychosocial, motor and language abilities. A new chapter on the executive functions has been added. Part III addresses assessment methodologies, both functional and standardized. The effects of impairment of cognitive abilities follow the same chapter headings as in Part II with summaries of the brain areas associated with each deficit.

The ultimate choice of assessments, which depends on the setting, the resources available, and the clinical reasoning of the therapist, is left to the reader. Finally, the list of references has been revised and expanded in response to the growth of cognitive rehabilitation in occupational therapy.

June Grieve

Acknowledgements

Firstly, my thanks to Jacqueline Adams and Tina Ashburner who encouraged me to write the first edition. In this second edition, my special thanks to four occupational therapists with clinical and training experience in neurology who have read, revised, edited and re-read particular topics with great patience. These areas are: the executive functions and dysexecutive syndrome by Fiona Adcock; attention and assessment by Susan Bennett; normal memory and memory problems by Jo Creighton; and task performance and dyspraxia by Thérèse Jackson.

Fiona Adcock developed the occupational therapy functional assessment of dysexecutive syndrome given in Chapter 15 based on Ylvisaker & Szekeres (1989) for clients with traumatic brain injury.

Jo Creighton devised and produced the original drawings in Parts I and II.

David Sanchez created the client/therapist figures in Part III.

Finally the task would not have been completed without the constant support of my family including the new arrivals, Alfie, Esme, Jack and Lola, whose cognitive development is a constant source of wonder to me.

Extracts from the Rivermead Perceptual Assessment Battery (Whiting *et al.*, 1985) are included by permission of the publishers, NFER-NELSON, Darville House, 2 Oxford Road East, Windsor, Berkshire, SL4 1DF. The extract from the Chessington Occupational Therapy Assessment Battery is included by permission of Nottingham Rehab, Ludlow Hill Road, West Bridgford, Nottingham, NG2 6HD. The extract from the Behavioural Inattention Test is included by per-mission of Thames Valley Test Company, 7–9 The Green, Flempton, Bury St Edmunds, Suffolk, IP28 6EL.

Part I

Theoretical Approaches to Perception and Cognition

Chapter 1   Introduction to Neuropsychology

Neuropsychology has grown out of the convergence of the medical science of neurology and psychology in the common study of the behavioural effects of brain damage. Impairments of brain function are associated with specific brain areas by studying groups of patients with common lesion sites and comparing them with normal subjects. Neuro-imaging studies use scanning techniques to identify the active brain areas during the performance of cognitive functions.

Cognitive psychology, since the 1950s, has studied the flow of information through the brain as a sequence of processing stages between input from the environment and output response in action and behaviour. Models of cognitive systems have been developed which are rigorously tested on normal subjects in the laboratory, and, more recently, in everyday life. In the 1970s, cognitive neuropsychology developed as a related discipline which applies the methodology of cognitive psychology to the study of impaired cognitive systems in patients with brain damage. The information processing approach to brain function has received further impetus from cognitive science which uses computer models to develop and test models of the cognitive systems.

The study of human brain function can be divided into two main approaches: the localization approach, based on function related to anatomical areas; and the holistic or information processing approach which focuses on the flow of information through the brain as a whole.

Localization

The localization approach interprets neurological deficits in terms of disruption of activity in specific brain areas, or the pathways between them. A simple analogy with a car would be that engine failure is due to damage of one of the parts of the engine, or to one of the electrical or mechanical connections between them. The features of the engine failure will depend on the part, or the connection, that is disrupted.

The phrenologists, in the early nineteenth century, were the first to suggest that the brain was divided into 'organs' or faculties with different intellectual and emotional functions, such as cautiousness, hope, self-esteem (Fig. 1.1). Gall, and his many followers, believed that a highly developed faculty indicated a correspondingly large area in the cerebral cortex, and that this was revealed in the head as a bump in the skull overlying it.

Later in the same century, the post-mortem examination of patients who had known deficits was used to indicate areas of the cerebral hemispheres that are concerned with the production of speech (Broca's area), and receptive aspects of speech and language (Wernicke's area) (Fig. 1.2). These discoveries were the first to localize language functions in the left hemisphere. At the turn of the century, neurologists described clusters of symptoms, known as syndromes, in patients with brain damage, based on detailed observation of their behaviour. An example is frontal lobe syndrome which is now known as dysexecutive syndrome. Later, the primary sensory and motor areas of the brain were identified by neurophysiologists in animal experiments and by neurosurgeons exploring the surface of the brain in epileptic patients to find the focus of the seizure.

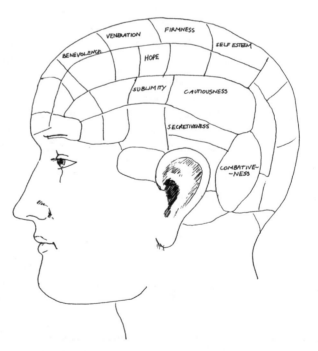

Fig. 1.1 Gall's phrenological map.

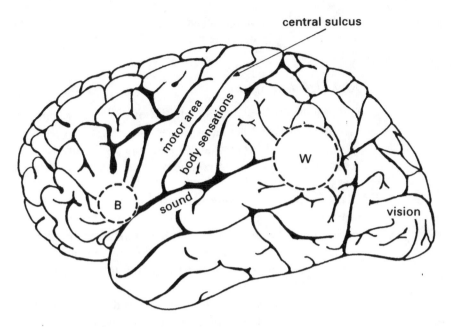

Fig. 1.2 Side view of the left cerebral hemisphere showing the primary motor and sensory areas. B – Broca's area, W – Wernicke's area.

Neuro-imaging techniques that identify lesions in the brain have been developed over recent years. Computerized tomography (CT scan) is now used routinely in the diagnosis of neurological disorders. Magnetic resonance imaging (MRI) locates soft tissue in the brain more clearly. Positron emission tomography (PET) scans indicate the areas of high levels of brain activity by sensing the local rate of blood flow from moment to moment. The MRI technique has also been adapted to measure physiological changes in the brain over time. This is known as fMRI. Functional imaging using PET and fMRI has advanced the localization approach to brain function as far as identifying some of the active sites when subjects perform cognitive tasks under controlled experimental conditions (Posner *et al.*, 1988). The methods of the neuro-imaging techniques are summarized in the glossary.

Neuropsychology has confirmed and extended the description of patterns of impairment that commonly occur together, known as syndromes. For example, the neglect syndrome is a failure to respond to stimuli in one side of external space. The neglected stimuli may be visual, auditory or tactile and the neglected space may be near or far. The presence of lesions in the right parietal lobe has been identified in patients with unilateral neglect. This provides evidence that spatial and attentional processing occurs in the right parietal lobe.

Right/left hemisphere

One outcome of localization studies of cerebral organization is the identification of differences in the capacity to process particular information in the right and left hemispheres. Figure 1.3 summarizes the anatomical description of the two hemispheres and their divisions into four lobes.

The dominant hemisphere, usually the left, tends to be larger and heavier than the non-dominant hemisphere. The inputs to the two sides from the senses, and from other brain areas and the spinal cord are largely the same, so any difference between the two must lie in their capacity to process different types of information.

- *The left hemisphere*, in most people, is dominant for all language functions: reading, writing, the understanding and the production of speech. These functions involve the processing of sequences; letter by letter, word by word and so on. The left hemisphere is also associated with sequences of action, which are the basis of most of our movements. For example, the actions of reach, grasp, lift, lower and release are performed in series in the activity of pouring water from a jug. The sequential processing involved in language, numeracy and movement means that the left hemisphere can be called the 'analyser'.

- *The right hemisphere* has a greater capacity to process visual and spatial information that cannot be described in words. The recognition of objects, the position of body parts during movement, and the spatial relationships of objects and landmarks in extra-personal space, are associated with the right hemisphere. The right hemisphere deals with wholes rather than parts and can be called the 'synthesizer' (Fig. 1.4a).

Comparisons of studies of patients after a cerebrovascular event (CVA) in either the right or the left hemisphere have been summarized by Heilman & Valenstein (1993) as follows: left CVAs have verbal communication difficulties including problems with receptive and expressive speech, and the sequencing and production of movements related to objects; and right CVAs have visuospatial problems including visual perceptual deficits, constructional problems and neglect of one side of space.

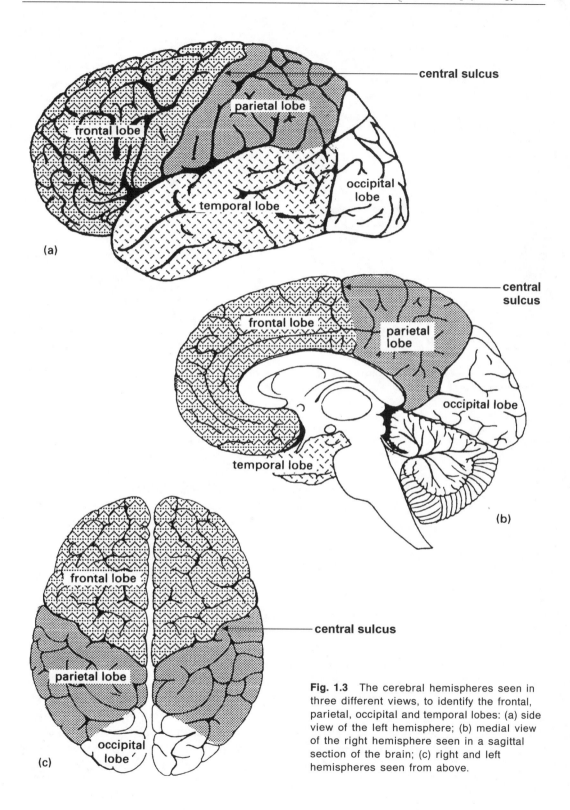

Fig. 1.3 The cerebral hemispheres seen in three different views, to identify the frontal, parietal, occipital and temporal lobes: (a) side view of the left hemisphere; (b) medial view of the right hemisphere seen in a sagittal section of the brain; (c) right and left hemispheres seen from above.

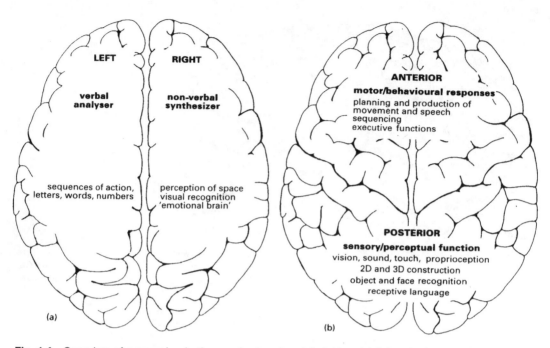

Fig. 1.4   Overview of processing in the cerebral cortex: (a) right and left hemispheres; (b) anterior and posterior divisions.

Differences in affective processing in the two hemispheres have led to the right hemisphere being called the 'emotional brain'. Left hemisphere lesion patients (right hemiplegics) often show feelings of anxiety and depression. Those with right hemisphere damage (left hemiplegics) may show indifference and denial of their disabilities, but they sometimes become depressed at a later stage in recovery as a result of loss of self-awareness and reduced sensitivity to others.

Anterior/posterior

The central sulcus (Fig. 1.3), divides each cerebral hemisphere into: a posterior division comprising the parietal, occipital and temporal lobes; and an anterior division, which is the frontal lobe.

- The *posterior* division receives projections from the ascending pathways of the spinal cord, and from the sense organs. Perceptual processing of these inputs occurs in the posterior division, including the visual and spatial processing of objects, faces and the landmarks we use to find our way around. The receptive aspects of language, such as understanding written and spoken words, are also part of the functions of the posterior cortex.

● The *anterior* division receives input from the posterior division and from lower brain centres. The motor centres for the performance of movement are located in the anterior division, as well as the output processing for the production of speech. Luria was one of the first neuropsychologists who suggested that the frontal lobes integrate all the components of movement and behaviour at the highest level (now translated and published in Luria, 1980). These high-level cognitive functions of planning, monitoring and modifying action and behaviour are now known as the executive functions (Fig. 1.4b).

The overview of cerebral organization into right/left and anterior/ posterior divisions provides a guide for the prediction of the possible functional problems that may result when the site of brain damage is known. However, patients with disruption in the same brain location can have different outcomes, depending on the extent of cerebral damage, and on the other brain areas that are involved.

Information processing

An alternative approach to the study of cognition is to consider the brain as a whole. The sensory information entering the brain from the environment under particular conditions can be defined and the output response in action and behaviour can be observed. Experiments are then devised to isolate and test the stages of processing between input and output. In this way a model of the stages operating in one component of cognition is developed. Each stage can be considered as groups of neurones firing together, but they may or may not be located in one particular brain area.

Historically, the holistic approach to brain function began as early as the nineteenth century when Fluorens, a French physiologist, opposed the localization view of the phrenologists. Based on animal experiments, he suggested that the cerebral cortex functions as a whole for all the mental processes of perception, cognition and intellect. Further strong support for the unitary function of the cerebral cortex was provided by Lashley in the 1930s. In learning studies in rats, he showed that functional deficits were related to the total size of damaged cortex, and not to the location of the damage.

Returning to the analogy of the car, it is the control units of the engine, or their operation by the driver, that determine the performance of the engine. The function of the separate engine parts may be a secondary factor. In the brain, the disruption of the coordination of processing stages may result in the emergence of the normally 'buried' lower-level activity. An example is perseveration, or repetition of action, seen in patients with interruption of the level of processing which controls the sequencing of action.

Stages/modules

In the models of cognitive systems developed in cognitive neuropsychology, each stage of processing is known as a module, and the flow of information from one module to the next is shown in an information processing diagram. If modules of cognitive processing are independent, it can be predicted that each can be selectively impaired. For example, if object recognition is impaired, the deficit may be at one of several different levels of processing: basic visual perception; visual structural description; semantic (meaning) representation; or lexical (name) representation (Fig. 1.5).

If a patient can use objects appropriately but cannot name them, this suggests there are independent modules for the knowledge of the names of familiar objects, and for the semantic representation of

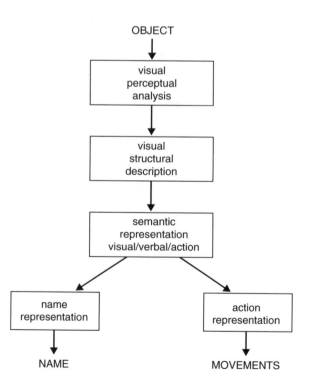

Fig. 1.5 Stages in processing, object naming and use.

the function of objects. In addition, if a different patient can name objects but cannot use them, this is further evidence for separate modules, known as double dissociation. Tests related to the individual modules in mental processing have been developed in cognitive neuropsychology and these are used to identify a deficit in a particular module. For example, tests may show that basic visual perception is intact, but if the patient cannot match all the forks in a drawer of mixed cutlery, this suggests impairment in forming the visual structural description of whole objects.

The modular approach to assessment can be used in occupational therapy to provide clues to the origin of cognitive impairment which can then be explored in the observation of functional tasks. The following list outlines the stages in the use of objects and the corresponding assessment.

Stage	Assessment
Visual perceptual analysis	Match colours, shapes, sizes
Structural description	Match objects
Semantic representation	Match objects by function
Action system	Perform the movements for the use of an object
Executive functions	Object use generalized to different environments

Perception and language have been described with modular models but some areas of cognition lend themselves less well to the modular approach. Both modular and non-modular components are included in the models of working memory and the executive system, where the modules are coordinated by a control unit.

Cognitive science has implemented computer programs in the study of cognitive systems. Parallel distributed processing models (or PDP) are developed from computer programs, known as networks, which learn and store different patterns of processing by repeated presentation of the same input. Networks may be compared to collections of neurones, but the nodes of the network do not have identical properties to synapses, so the analogy can be misleading. The changes in the output of the system when a part of a network is degraded can simulate the effects of lesion of a brain area.

A purely modular-based description of the operation of all the cognitive systems is too simplistic. In Part II, models of the stages of processing in some perceptual and cognitive abilities will be presented where they provide a basis for the development of assessment procedures.

References

Heilman, K. M. & Valenstein, E. (1993) *Clinical Neuropsychology*. New York: Oxford University Press.

Luria, A. R. (1980) *Higher Cortical Functions in Man*. New York: Basic Books.

Posner, M. I., Peterson, S. E., Fox, P. T. & Raichle, M. E. (1988) Localization of cognitive processes. *Science* **240**, 1627–31.

Further reading

Hampson, P. J. & Morris, P. E. (1996) Understanding cognition. In *Cognitive Neuropsychology*, pp. 296–326. Oxford: Blackwell Publishers Ltd.

Rothi, I. & Bruce, V. (1995) *Perception and Representation*. Buckingham: Open University Press.

Chapter 2　Perception and Cognition in Human Occupation

From moment to moment all the senses – vision, sound, smell, touch, pain and proprioception – pick up information from the world around us, and from inside the body. Perception is the processing in the brain that transforms all this information into our immediate experience of the world. We are usually unaware of perception, and it is very fast acting. However, perception is not simply based on the input that the brain receives via the senses. Our expectations and our past experience have an active influence on perception. Also, what we perceive may be changed by the context in which we see it.

Cognition comprises all the mental processes that allow us perform meaningful actions and behaviour. Learning, recognition, memory and attention are all parts of the cognitive system, as well as the ability to plan, monitor and adapt to the changing information in the environment. The parts of the complex cognitive system operate to achieve a common goal and several components may be involved in one functional activity. For example, in making a phone call, finding the number, remembering it long enough to dial, and then speaking and listening, each has different cognitive demands (Fig. 2.1).

Theories of perception

Perception can be defined as: making sense of the senses; or the ability to process and interpret information from the environment to make a meaningful whole. There have been two main approaches to the investigation of perception in cognitive psychology.

'Bottom-up' theories

These theories begin with the detailed analysis of the sensory input, and proceed to the integration of all this information with our stored knowledge of past experience. These are known as 'bottom-up' or

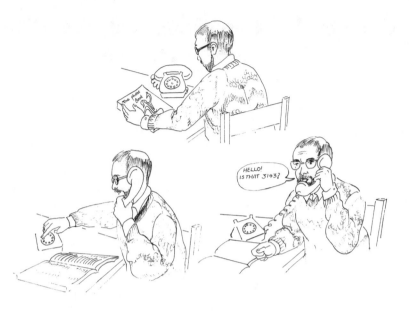

Fig. 2.1 Stages in using the telephone.

'data-driven' theories which consider that perception is driven by the sensory information that is available from the environment.

If perception depended only on bottom-up processing of all the input from the senses, the capacity of the brain would be exceeded. Also the input from the retinal image may be too ambiguous to form the basis of our visual perception of the world around us.

'Top-down' theories

Another set of theories of perception begin with the stored knowledge of past experience, and consider how this is used to make sense of the changing sensory input entering the brain. These are known as 'top-down' or 'concept-driven' theories. Detailed analysis of all the sensory input is not required, and this means there is economy of the processing demands.

Evidence for top-down processing is the way we can make sense of ambiguous information. In vision, the same input to the retina can be perceived in different ways (Fig. 2.2).

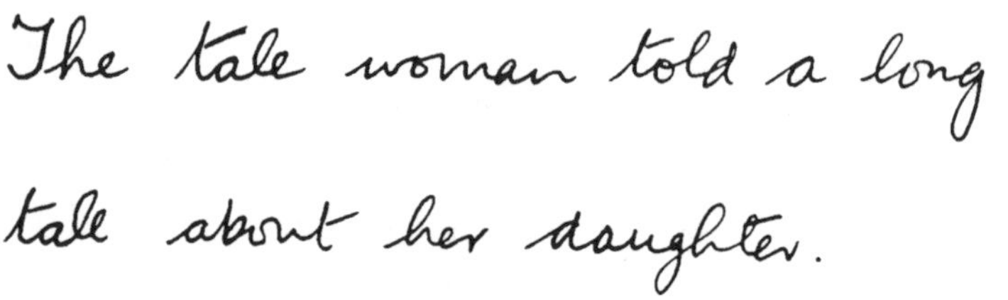

The tale woman told a long

tale about her daughter.

Fig. 2.2 Top-down processing in perception.

In this sentence, two of the words present the same pattern to the retina, but one is perceived as 'tall' and the other as 'tale'.

In sound, the same speech output can be perceived as different. Read aloud the following two sentences:

'That noise makes me want to scream.'
'Here is some vanilla ice cream.'

The same sensory input can only be perceived in different ways if it is influenced by our stored knowledge, and by the context in which it is presented.

It is generally agreed in psychology that perception depends on both bottom-up and top-down processing. We interpret what the senses pick up by integration with past experience. The link between perception and learned experience allows us to adapt behaviour appropriately in response to changes in the sensory input. The functional problems in patients who have no sensory loss may originate in disordered perception or in the retrieval of stored knowledge related to the task.

Normal perception is so spontaneous and automatic that it is difficult to understand the experience of impaired perception in a patient with brain damage. While the effects of altered sensory input can be experienced by blindfolding our eyes or plugging our ears, understanding disordered perception is more problematic. When the sensory input is confusing, we have to make an effort to find a solution. The responses of a group of people to looking at an ambiguous figure illustrate this (Fig. 2.3).

Some may 'see' it as an old woman, and some may 'see' it as a young woman. After a time, many will 'see' it as either one or the other, or neither and say 'I will see it when I believe it'. It is these exercises that begin to make us realize what it is like for patients with perceptual problems. For them, looking at a cup and saucer may require the effort we needed to find a solution to the ambiguous figure.

Cognition: one system or many?

Cognition is a complex and dynamic system of interrelated parts which allows us to organize and use knowledge in order to function in the environment in which we live. New information entering the system is organized and classified. Old information is retrieved for

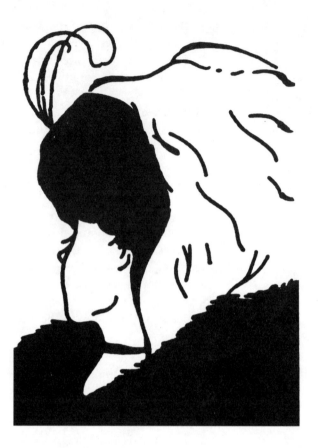

Fig. 2.3 Ambiguous figure.

the interpretation of the current processing. The output response may be action, or decision-making, or storage of information for future use.

The early stages in cognitive processing include visual and auditory perceptual analysis of the sensory input, with attention directing the processing to particular stimuli. After the semantic stage of processing (see Chapter 1), the output response is activated if a routine task is being performed, and the task proceeds automatically with a low level of sustained attention. An example of this occurs when we get into our own car and put in the ignition key. This activates the sequence of movements for getting into gear, releasing the brake and pressing the accelerator. Driving proceeds automatically until a new set of actions is triggered by a change, such as a bend in the road or traffic lights. Routine tasks in daily living are performed automatically with a low level of control. When our environment changes, such as moving house or starting a new job, a higher level of cognitive processing is demanded while we respond to novel situations. After a time, new routines are established in memory.

Non-routine tasks require an attention control unit which focuses on the relevant processing level over time. For example, in working memory a central attention system interacts with two separate modules for short-term processing of visual or verbal information from the environment. When we perform two tasks at a time, switching of attention occurs from one task to the other. Washing-up and listening to a play on the radio, for example, are dual tasks that can be performed within the normal limits of attention capacity.

Cognition is involved in the planning of actions and behaviours to reach a goal, for example to visit a friend on her birthday. Decision-making, and prospective memory for future actions, are required at the start of the journey (go by car, or bus, or walk?; go on the right day). If the route we choose is blocked by road works on that day, the executive processing is recruited to modify the plan and monitor the progress until we get there. Finding the way also involves spatial processing of the features of the environment, and of our bodies in relation to the route we follow.

Stored knowledge about the world is only one part of memory. Skilled actions depend on the activation of stored procedures for their performance. These procedures are developed and improved with time so that we become more proficient at activities such as touch-typing or playing a musical instrument.

The cognitive system normally functions as a whole, but it is necessary to make divisions, sometimes called subsystems, in order to understand the way the component parts operate. The identification of a deficit in a cognitive subsystem may provide a basis for explaining occupational dysfunction. Also the observation of functional activities is enhanced by an understanding of the underlying cognitive skills that support effective performance. There is no single way of dividing the cognitive system. The organization of the chapters in this book reflects the cognitive abilities that are the concern of the occupational therapist in the assessment and treatment of patients with neurological problems. In Parts II and III the components of perception and cognition will be grouped under the headings:

(1) *Visual perception*:
    (a) basic visual perception, object and face recognition
(2) *Spatial abilities*:
    (a) scanning of space
    (b) body scheme, constructional praxis, topographical orientation

(3) *Attention*:
   (a) alertness and arousal
   (b) sustained, selective and divided attention
(4) *Memory*:
   (a) working memory
   (b) long-term memory – procedural, declarative, prospective
   (c) everyday memory
(5) *Task performance*:
   (a) action schemas
   (b) models of praxis
(6) *Executive functions*:
   (a) routine and non-routine action and behaviour
   (b) flexible problem-solving
   (c) self-reflectiveness.

The language system, a major component of cognition, is not included. Communication with speech and language therapists should be facilitated by the modular approach to some of the cognitive abilities presented in Part II.

Neurological conditions

Deficits in perception and cognition occur in:

- cerebral vascular accident or stroke
- traumatic brain injury
- viral encephalitis
- multiple sclerosis
- cerebral tumours
- anoxia resulting from carbon monoxide poisoning or accidents in anaesthesia
- Parkinson's disease
- Korsakoff's syndrome

The changes in the dementias and Alzheimer's disease are complicated by global cognitive and intellectual deterioration. A comprehensive account of neuropsychological studies of the degenerative diseases, including the psychosocial and behavioural changes, can be found in Knight (1992). Some patients may have more than one neurological disorder, for example Parkinson's disease complicated by a stroke.

The brain damage resulting from a specific neurological disorder has variable effects on the function of the individual patient. The variation may be due to:

- the complex organization of the brain
- the pathology of the disease
- pre-morbid personality
- age, culture, and social background.

Many of the studies in neuropsychology have investigated perception and cognition in stroke patients, where the deficits are circumscribed, due to the focal nature of the lesion. A group study of 227 stroke patients three months post-admission compared with 240 control subjects found that the components of cognition that were most likely to be impaired were: memory, orientation, language and attention (Tatemichi *et al.*, 1994). Over recent years there have been an increasing number of studies of the cognitive problems resulting from traumatic brain injury (TBI) when multiple lesions occur. If the frontal lobes are involved in TBI, executive deficits may affect all occupational performance with the exception of some well-learned routine tasks.

The number of people with brain damage due to injury, disease or degenerative conditions living in the community is increasing. In the home environment, the assessment of perceptual and cognitive abilities can be carried out in a realistic setting with added information from family and carers.

References

Knight, R. G. (1992) *The Neuropsychology of Degenerative Diseases.* New Jersey: Lawrence Erlbaum.

Tatemichi, T. K., Desmond, D. W., Stern, Y., Park, M., Sano, M. & Bagiella, E. (1994) Cognitive impairment after stroke. *Journal of Neurology, Neurosurgery and Psychiatry* **57**, 202–207.

Further reading

Green, J. & Hicks, C. (1984) *Basic Cognitive Processes.* Milton Keynes: Open University Press.

Smyth, M. M., Morris, P. E., Levy, P. & Ellis, A. (1994) *Cognition in Action.* London: Lawrence Erlbaum.

Part II

Perceptual and Cognitive Abilities

Chapter 3 Visual Perception, Object and Face Recognition

Visual perception gives meaning to all the information entering the eyes. Our perception of the complex visual world is largely automatic. While the information entering the eyes is constantly varying, we perceive individual objects, people and landmarks as the same whatever their position, illumination or distance from us. Vision plays a major role in the total perception of the environment and the brain has a larger area of cortex devoted to the processing of vision than any of the other senses.

The adaptability of visual perception has been dramatically illustrated in an experiment when subjects wore spectacles with inverting lenses. After several days, the subjects had adapted to the upside-down view of the world. They were able to move around normally, and perform all activities of daily living. The ability to instantly recognize the features of the visual environment seems to be so easy that it may be difficult to appreciate how many complex processes are involved. As we look out of the window, we can decide where a house ends and a tree begins, if they are overlapping. Drawing or painting a scene makes us aware of clues about depth and distance (Fig. 3.1).

Looking around a room, each object is isolated from its background, and from other objects around it. The same object is recognized irrespective of the angle from which we are looking at it, and its distance from us. In using objects, the visual recognition is associated with their meaning and their function when we use them. In social interaction we need to recognize faces and associate them with the names of the people we know. As we move about, landmarks are recognized and obstructions are avoided. Complex perceptual and cognitive processing is involved in all of these situations.

So what features of the retinal image are processed by the brain, and how are features transformed into our perception of the three-dimensional world? The impressionist painters were able to create three-dimensional scenes from flat planes of colour on a canvas. In psychology, several different approaches have been used to study

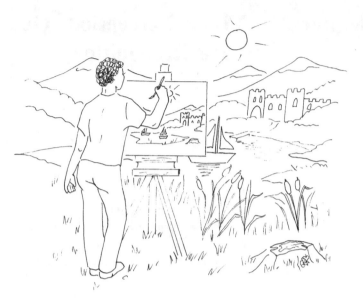

Fig. 3.1 Painting a scene.

how the brain analyses the retinal image, and to describe the processes that lead to the recognition of objects and faces.

Basic visual perception

The perceptual analysis of an object involves the integration of several basic features. Sensory information about the colour of objects, their surface texture, and the direction of lines and edges in the surroundings are all parts of visual perception. Outlines are isolated from their background, and an object is seen as the same in different views. The basic features which contribute to the perceptual analysis of an object will now be considered.

Colour

Colour in the visual environment gives added meaning. In child development, the toddler learns that the colour and the form of particular objects are associated with their function. Even in different lighting conditions, familiar objects do not change their colour. Similar items that may be in different colours, for example coins, or food in jars, depend on colour discrimination for identification.

Colour perception is different from colour blindness, which is a retinal defect. When there is loss of colour perception, the world is seen as shades of grey, and vision is reported as 'not clear' even though visual acuity is normal.

Selective impairment of colour and shape has been described in patients with cerebral damage. This suggests that in early visual processing, colour is processed separately from shape and depth.

Depth

Depth perception comes partly from the difference in the image of an object received by the retina of each eye. There are, however, other clues in the visual field which provide information about depth. If one object partly obscures another, the complete object is perceived to be nearer. When similar objects appear to be of different sizes, the larger ones are perceived to be nearer, and the smaller ones further away. Parallel lines appear to converge, and textures become finer, in the distance. The mugs on a tray in Fig. 3.2 illustrate these clues to depth perception.

Movement can also be part of depth perception. Sitting in a moving car, nearby features of the visual scene, such as telegraph poles, appear to move by quickly, while distant trees appear to move slowly. The perception of depth is also basic to spatial abilities, discussed in Chapter 4.

Figure ground

The Gestalt psychologists in the 1920s first proposed that perception is organized to produce 'good form'. They introduced the term 'figure ground'. In the visual world, we perceive whole objects set in a background. All the items and objects we use must be isolated from

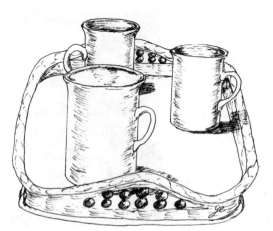

Fig. 3.2 Clues for depth perception.

the surfaces they lie on, and from other objects that overlap them. The three mugs shown in Fig. 3.2 form the 'figure', and the tray is the 'ground'.

Activity _____

Look around the room you are in and count the number of objects you can see. Then count how many of the objects are overlapped by other objects. Move to the other side of the room where you see different views of the same objects and at different distances. Note the shadows cast by the light from the window or lamp falling on the objects, and how the textures of surfaces change in the distance.

Visual perception segments the environment into what is figure and what is ground. It is the grouping together of the elements of colour, form and depth that produces the figure and separates it from the ground. Many visual illusions are pictures where the figure and the ground can be exchanged. Figure 3.3 can be perceived as a vase or two faces in silhouette, depending on whether the black area or the white area respectively is seen as the ground.

A patient with impairment of figure ground has difficulty in picking out objects when they are surrounded by others, for example cutlery in a drawer, or an item of clothing lying on a bed.

Form constancy

Objects are seen as the same size, shape and location, even though there are variations in their image on the retina. This is known as

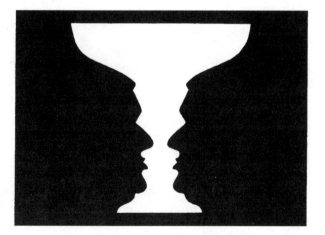

Fig. 3.3 Figure ground – two different interpretations.

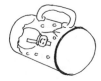

Fig. 3.4 Object constancy – object seen in different orientations.

perceptual constancy, and without it the visual world would be very confusing.

The table I write on appears the same size when I stand one metre away, or six metres across the room. As I move about the room, I do not see the table moving about, even though the image of the table on my retina is changing. If I tilt my head to one side, the retinal image again changes, but the table appears the same.

Object constancy allows us to identify the same object when it is seen in different views and orientations (Fig. 3.4). If we are shown an unfamiliar object, we can still identify it as the same object when we see it from above, from below, at an angle, and so on.

Size discrimination is part of form constancy. We can distinguish the same shape, seen in different sizes, from other shapes or objects.

In summary, the basic strands of visual processing of colour, shape, figure ground and form constancy combine to complete the perceptual processing that leads to the mental representation of an object in all views. Evidence from studies of patients with right or left hemisphere lesion suggest that visual perceptual analysis occurs in the right hemisphere. In right hemisphere lesions (left hemiplegia), the inability to complete this visual perceptual analysis is the basis of poor object recognition.

Visual object recognition

The recognition of objects depends on the integration of visual perception with stored knowledge of known objects. In task performance, the output of recognition processes must then be integrated with knowledge of their meaning and function. This in turn allows us to perform the correct movements for their use.

Object recognition has been studied in cognitive psychology using: laboratory experiments asking subjects to respond to different types of visual information; computer systems designed to operate on visual images; and assessment of patients with visual recognition problems to identify the impaired modules.

Modular approaches to object recognition have described the sequence of stages of processing from the retinal image to the recognition of objects. Top-down approaches, on the other hand, have emphasized the importance of contextual information in object recognition. Textures, surfaces and lines in the visual environment give meaning to what we see, and these are interpreted in the context of the changing scene around us. Gibson (1979) proposed that surfaces and objects 'afford' action. The affordance of an object is what it offers as a possibility for action. A handle affords grasping, the shape of a jug affords tipping (Fig. 3.5). Some patients who have poor semantic knowledge of the meaning of objects can use them by activating the action system by a direct route from perception to action (Riddoch & Humphreys, 1987).

Contextual information is important in visual recognition, so that functional assessments in occupational therapy are facilitated in the patient's familiar environment, and with objects previously known to them.

A functional model for object recognition (Ellis & Young, 1988) based on the methods of cognitive neuropsychology is given in Fig. 3.6.

- The viewer-centred representation is the output of early visual perceptual processing. This level is intact if the patient can copy line drawings and match objects.
- The object-centred representation is the mental processing of objects which can be recognized in any view. This level can be assessed by matching and recognition of the same object in different views.
- The object recognition units are stored descriptions of known objects in memory. The outputs from the viewer-centred and the object-centred representations are compared with these stored descriptions for recognition of a known object.
- In the semantic system, the output from visual recognition processing accesses stored knowledge of the meaning and function of objects. The semantic representation may also be accessed from tactile input, or from a verbal description of an object. If there is no deficit in the semantic system, objects can be matched by function, and can be used appropriately.

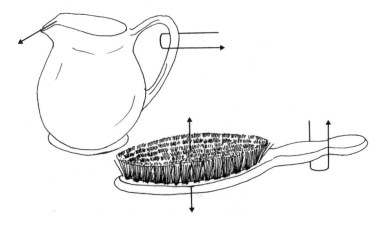

Fig. 3.5 Direct perception and action: jug 'affords' grasping and tipping; brush 'affords' grasping and moving up and down.

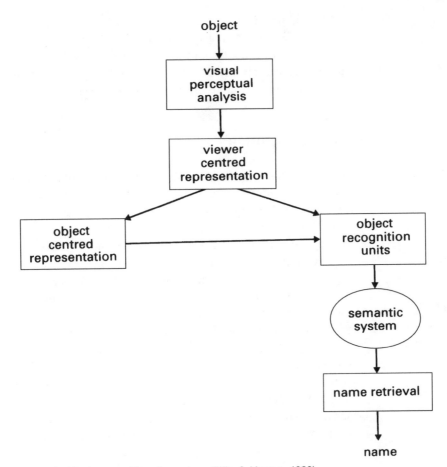

Fig. 3.6   Model of object recognition (based on Ellis & Young, 1988).

- The name of an object is achieved by access to the lexicon of the names of known objects. Interruption at this level means that an object may be recognized and used, but cannot be named.

Output from the semantic system must also access the action system to activate the movements that are associated with the use of the object. This output level is considered in relation to task performance in Chapter 7.

There is considerable evidence for the separation of: structural; semantic and naming levels; of processing in object recognition, although some cross-modular processing (known as cascade) may occur. The three levels provide a basis for identifying the level of impairment, which can then be related to the observation of functional performance with objects.

It is important to appreciate that problems in the use of objects can arise for a variety of reasons. Toglia (1989) suggests that functional assessment in occupational therapy should include: the effects of the number of objects present; the spatial arrangement of the objects; the complexity of the task; and the environment.

Face recognition

The recognition of faces is not the same as recognition of objects; a face offers so much more information than an object. In a face we are presented with expressions of emotion, and with speech, both of which are unique to that person. We integrate this with other information, for example age, sex, occupation and behaviour.

In common with objects, a face can be processed as a visual structure, recognized as a face when seen from different views, and we know whether a face is familiar or not. The identity of a known person, however, can be made just from the sound of his/her voice, or from a fleeting glimpse in a crowd.

The question 'What is unique about the processing of faces compared with objects?' has been studied in cognitive psychology. If there are differences, they are in the processing of facial expression and facial speech (lip-reading). There has been some support for a separate area of cortex for faces only. A very young baby makes movements of the eyes and head to follow the face of someone in his or her view, and may copy their facial expressions. However, like sucking, this early processing may be replaced by others in later stages of development.

A model of the processing of faces described by Bruce & Young (1986) is based on single case studies of patients with problems in recognizing familiar faces (Fig. 3.7). A number of modules are linked in series or in parallel.

- The visual perceptual analysis of a face discriminates the visual elements of a face; the eyes, the nose, the mouth and so on. A patient who has a disruption at this early stage is unable to distinguish these basic features of a face, and he or she is likely to have more widespread perceptual difficulties.
- The viewer-centred description distinguishes a face as different from objects and other items. This is shown by the ability to match faces.
- The face recognition units allow the identification of a known face but not a particular person. This level is based on the ability to

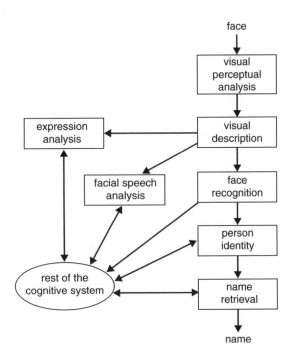

Fig. 3.7 Model of face recognition (based on Bruce & Young, 1986).

discriminate the faces of unfamiliar people, and to match different views of an unfamiliar face.

- The person identity nodes are stored knowledge of the identity of particular known people. Here the output from the face recognition units activates the representation of a known person.
- Facial expressions and facial speech access the person identity nodes via the semantic system. Bruce and Young suggest that access to this final recognition stage is also via other semantic knowledge about known people, such as family relationships or occupation.
- Name retrieval is the final stage of processing in this model. Disruption at this stage means that the person has been identified but cannot be named.

Severe problems with face recognition are rare and may occur in stroke patients with bilateral posterior lesions, or in patients with multiple posterior lesions following traumatic brain injury. The inability to learn the names of hospital staff is usually a memory problem. Loss of face recognition for close family and friends is distressing. Advice to relatives and friends on the importance of the voice and facial expressions can reduce the stress for the patient.

Summary

(1)   Visual perception organizes the visual environment into a mean-
      ingful whole. Basic visual perception includes colour, depth, the
      isolation of shapes and objects from their background (figure
      ground), and recognition of them in a variety of viewing
      conditions (form constancy).
(2)   Some theories of visual perception have considered bottom-up
      processing from the analysis of the retinal image to recognition.
      Other top-down processing theories emphasize the importance
      of past experience to make sense of the information in the
      sensory input in terms of expectations about the visual world.
(3)   Modular models of object recognition show the relationship of
      three main stages of processing in series: structural description;
      semantic representation of the meaning and use of objects; and
      name representation for object naming. Each of these levels can
      be selectively impaired.
(4)   A model of face recognition follows similar stages of processing
      to objects, with additional modules for facial expression and
      facial speech processed in parallel.

References

Bruce, V. & Young, A. W. (1986) Understanding face recognition. *Journal of
    Psychology* **77**, 305–27.
Ellis, A. W. & Young, A. W. (1988) *Human Cognitive Neuropsychology*. London:
    Lawrence Erlbaum.
Gibson, J. J. (1979) *The Ecological Approach to Visual Perception*. Boston:
    Houghton Miffin.
Riddoch, M. J. & Humphreys, G. W. (1987) Visual object processing in a case of
    optic aphasia: a case of semantic access agnosia. *Cognitive Neuropsychology* **4**,
    131–85.
Toglia, J. P. (1989) Visual perception of objects. An approach to assessment and
    intervention. *American Journal of Occupational Therapy* **43**, 587–95.

Further reading

Humphreys, G. W. & Riddoch, M. J. (1987) *To See or Not to See. A Case Study
    of Visual Agnosia*. London: Lawrence Erlbaum.
Rothi, I. & Bruce, V. (1995) *Perception and Representation: Current Issues*.
    Buckingham: Open University Press.

Chapter 4   Spatial Abilities

In the visual exploration of space ahead we scan the area of space offered by the visual field of both eyes, and beyond this by moving the eyes and the head. Once an object or a surface has been located, the spatial analysis of its relation to other objects around, and to ourselves, is required. All functional activities have a spatial component, especially constructional tasks that need the assembly of parts into a whole. A mental representation of body parts and their relative position in space must be integrated with objects in the environment in order to use them. On a larger scale, the spatial relations of buildings and landmarks are important in finding our way around on foot, on a bicycle or in a car. We need to discriminate right and left, and to be able to mentally rotate a pathway to follow it in different directions (Fig. 4.1). The building up of a mental spatial map of

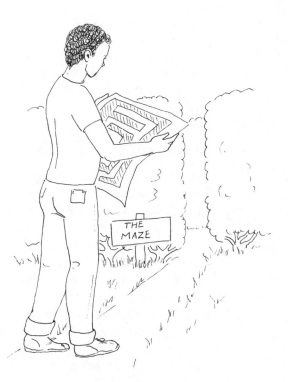

Fig. 4.1 Map of a maze.

familiar surroundings may change the task of route-finding into one of spatial memory.

Spatial processing as a part of everyday functioning has not been investigated to the same extent as other elements of perception. One reason may be the complex nature of spatial perception. A wide range of discrete abilities are involved in the exploration of different areas of space.

This chapter will start with the scanning movements of the eyes which are crucial for the processing of all visual and spatial information. This will be followed by three different spatial components: body scheme – the processing of the position and relationships of body parts; constructional praxis – the integration of spatial and motor elements when parts are assembled into a whole; and topographical orientation – the movement of the whole body in the environment. The perceptual disorder of unilateral neglect is often included with visuospatial processing. There is, however, a major attention component to this deficit and unilateral neglect will be included in Chapters 5 and 12.

Scanning of space

The area of the visual field ahead determines the space that is available for visual and spatial perception without moving the eyes. The visual field is like a window to the visual world. The view through the window can be scanned by movements of the eyes. Movements of the head take the window to different positions around the scene ahead, and this increases the area that can be scanned.

Visual field

If we look straight ahead, the area of the visual world that is visible out of each eye is known as the visual field for that eye. The right and left visual fields overlap in the midline, so that some light from each visual field reaches the retina of both eyes.

'Blind areas' appear in the visual fields, as a result of disruption at any level in the visual pathway from the retina to the occipital cortex itself. The opportunity for visuospatial perception without head movement is then restricted.

The visual pathway from one visual field reaches the occipital lobe of the opposite side (Fig. 4.2). Follow the projection from the left visual field to the inner nasal half of the left retina, and to the outer temporal half of the right retina. Now continue the same path (shown

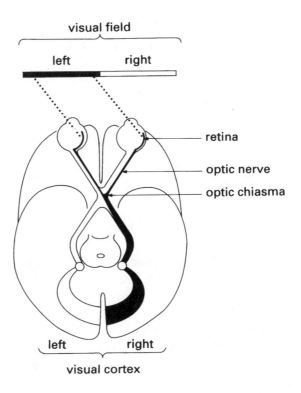

Fig. 4.2 Visual field and the visual pathway. Information from one visual field enters both eyes and reaches the visual cortex of the opposite side.

in black) on to the optic chiasma, and then to the right occipital lobe. You can now appreciate how damage to one occipital lobe can produce 'blind areas' in half the visual field of each eye.

Patients with posterior lesions due to a cerebrovascular accident or traumatic brain injury may have 'blind areas' of varying size and position in the visual fields, depending on the particular level of disruption of the visual pathway. These patients usually compensate for this defect successfully by movements of the head.

An estimate of the area of the normal visual field can be shown in the following way:

Activity

Stand behind a partner and ask him or her to focus on an object straight ahead. Place your fingers at different positions to either side, above and below, and ask your partner to report when the fingers are seen.

Experience of how loss of part of the visual fields affects perception can be gained by the following:

Activity _____

Cut out quarters or halves of a circle in black paper. Stick pairs of corresponding shapes onto the inner half of one lens and the outer half of the other lens of a pair of spectacles. Wear these spectacles while you walk about, write, read and make a cup of coffee.

Eye movements

Most of the time, we scan the space around by moving the eyes and the head. The extraocular muscles, which execute the movements of the eyes, are innervated by three cranial nerves originating in the brain stem. The control of eye movements associated with the exploration of space includes projections to the brain stem from cortical areas in the frontal and occipital lobes. There are two types of eye movement: pursuit and saccades.

- The *pursuit* type of eye movement is a slow movement of the eyes at the same rate as a moving image in order to keep the image on the central part of the retina. In many sports activities and in computer games the eyes must follow a ball or figure as it moves towards a target. Pursuit movements of the eyes originate in the occipital lobes.
- *Saccadic* eye movements are made in scanning a static display. In reading, the fixation of the eyes on a group of words is alternated with rapid eye movements known as saccades to the next group of words along the line. In scanning a larger area such as a picture, the eyes first make long saccades from the centre to the periphery, followed by shorter and shorter saccades to fixate on the detail of the picture. Saccadic movements of the eyes originate in the supplementary motor area of the frontal lobes which activate the brain stem nuclei to produce a rapid movement of the eyes to the opposite side.

Saccadic and pursuit eye movements can be seen in the following way:

Activity _____

(1) Ask a partner to move his or her eyes in a straight line from left to right. You will see the eyes make saccades and fixations as the imaginary line is scanned. Alternatively, position yourself so that you can watch the eyes of someone

reading a book. You will see alternate saccades and fixations as the eyes scan the lines of the page.

(2) Ask a partner to fixate on the tip of a pencil which you move across from left to right. Observe how the eyes move slowly as they follow the target.

As we move around, the head moves with each step. Also in talking to other people, we move the head to express feelings. In these conditions a stable gaze is maintained by small eye movements activated by the vestibular system responding to movements of the head.

Adequate scanning of the space around us depends on: the area of the visual field in both eyes; and oculomotor control of the position of the eyes to keep the image of items on the central part of the retina.

Fractionation of space

The body movements made in the different areas of space are related to the type of activities performed there. These can be divided into: manipulation of objects in contact with the body; reaching and grasping objects away from the body; and locomotion or moving the whole body in the environment (Fig. 4.3).

For purposes of description, three areas of space around the body have been described which relate to these functional movements:

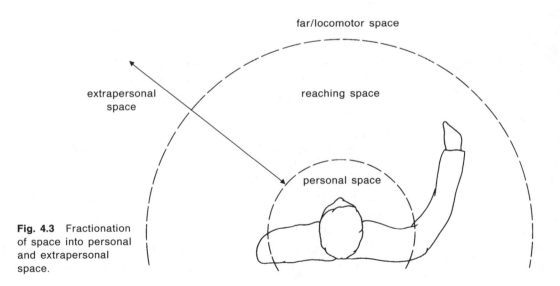

Fig. 4.3 Fractionation of space into personal and extrapersonal space.

- personal space
- extrapersonal/reaching space
- extrapersonal/far space, which may be called locomotor space.

There is evidence for selective processing in these three areas of space based on studies of unilateral neglect (see Chapter 5).

Body scheme

Body scheme is the mental representation of the parts of the body and the relative position of the body parts in space.

Knowledge of the spatial relationship between the different body segments is crucial in all movement. The sensory input from vision and proprioception must be integrated into a scheme of the whole body. Impairment of body scheme affects the execution of voluntary movement and the quality of task performance.

Sirigu *et al.* (1991) suggest that several different representations are incorporated into body knowledge processing:

- the lexical (name) and semantic (function) representation of each body part, e.g. the hand is used for grasping;
- a structural description of the position of each part in the body, e.g. the hand is at the end of the upper limb;
- the spatiotemporal representation of the changing positions of body parts.

The representation of body scheme in more than one form means that there are various features of body scheme disorder. There is some support for the distinction of body image from body scheme, although the use of these terms in the literature is confusing. Body image combines body scheme with emotional and environmental inputs which produce a representation of our own body in visual imagery. This representation is not the same as the exact physical appearance of our own body. When normal subjects are asked to draw a picture of themselves, the relative sizes of some body features may be larger or smaller than they really are.

In a review of body scheme disorders and their assessment, Corbett & Shah (1996) suggest that more definitive studies are needed of how body scheme disorders affect function. The incidence of body scheme disorder in stroke patients and its adverse effect on function makes body scheme a priority for research in occupational therapy.

Body scheme plays a major role in all the activities in personal care which take place in personal space (Fig. 4.3). In washing, toileting and dressing, the arms and hands are used to manipulate objects and items of clothing in contact with the parts of the body. A crucial element in negotiating stairs and kerbs is the knowledge of the distance moved by the lower limbs at each step. Visually impaired people rely more heavily on proprioception and body scheme to estimate the depth of stairs.

Constructional praxis

Constructional praxis is the ability to perform the movements to organize single units into a two- or three-dimensional whole.

In drawing, the parts must be placed into the correct relative positions of the whole in two dimensions on the page, which may be easy when copying a two-dimensional figure. A more difficult spatial operation is involved when drawing a figure or an item from memory, since the three-dimensional subject in visual imagery must be converted into a two-dimensional drawing.

Constructional praxis in three dimensions has a greater relevance to everyday tasks. In the performance of activities in reaching space the location of objects in the environment must be integrated with the extent and direction of movement. This demands the knowledge of both the spatial orientation of the moving body segments and of the objects being manipulated, particularly when there is a constructional element to the task. There is a constructional component in meal preparation, for example making a sandwich and setting the table, and in dressing. Component parts of equipment used at work and at home have to be assembled into a particular three-dimensional arrangement. There is a large spatial component to maintenance and repair tasks, such as fixing a car engine or a lawn mower (Fig. 4.4).

The investigation of constructional praxis in neuropsychology has centred around analysis of the drawings or block designs executed by patients with right or left hemisphere lesion. One of the difficulties in the assessment of spatial processing is in isolating the spatial component from the motor output to execute the task. In an early study by Warrington *et al.* (1966), the drawings made by patients with right hemisphere lesion showed disruption of the spatial arrangement of the parts. The left hemisphere lesion patients produced simplified drawings, which could be accounted for by poor execution of the movements required. If drawings are to be used for the assessment of

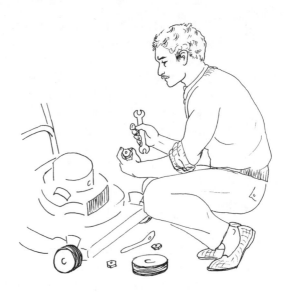

Fig. 4.4   Constructional ability.

constructional deficits there is a need to develop clear descriptions to distinguish the types of errors produced.

In patients with left hemisphere lesion (right hemiplegia), motor deficits pose an additional problem in devising tests of constructional praxis when the non-dominant hand may have to be used. In a patient with frontal lobe damage, the presence of executive deficits may affect the results, particularly using the non-dominant hand (see Chapter 8).

Copying figures and constructing block designs are simple screening tests that are quick and easy. They may provide useful predictors of problems in functional tasks.

Topographical orientation

Our ability to move from place to place in the three-dimensional world depends on a complex navigation system which operates on large-scale spatial knowledge. The topographical environment surrounds us and it is viewed from many different perspectives. As we explore our surroundings, spatial working memory holds information from the environment for a few seconds at a time (see Chapter 6), and retrieves spatial information from long-term memory for planning the sequence of movements along the way. Attention and visual recognition of landmarks are basic to route-finding, while visual and tactile perception may offer additional information.

Topographical orientation is a cognitive ability which has three stages of knowledge acquisition:

(1) Stored knowledge of known landmarks and their spatial rela-
     tion to both the body and to each other. This stage is known
     as egocentric or body centred. It includes the ability to judge
     proximity, depth, and the orientation of landmarks with respect
     to ourselves.
(2) Route knowledge that connects the landmarks in a sequential
     order.
(3) Representations of combined landmarks and routes, which may
     be called cognitive mapping. This stage is known as allocentric
     or environment centred. It is independent of where we are or our
     orientation in space.

These three stages occur in series in child development. The young
child first learns to recognize 'my house', 'my road', and 'Mary's door'
at the crèche. Next he/she knows where to turn the corner on familiar
routes. The ability to find different paths between two known places,
or to find new routes, develops later.

We experience these stages when we move to a new home, or arrive
at college or a new place of work. We start by learning the landmarks
on the way to the local supermarket, the occupational therapy (OT)
department or the library. These short routes are then expanded and
extended as we explore other parts of the area. The final stage is when
we can find the way between two locations by different routes. One
route is better than another when it is raining, or if you need wheelchair access for a patient. This requires the development of allocentric
knowledge constructed from the combination of landmarks and
routes. Moving around then becomes automatic.

If we get lost, we use visual or verbal strategies by looking at a map
or asking the way. Some people say that they have no sense of
direction, and others say that they cannot read maps. This highlights
the individual differences in the strategies we use in finding our way
around. The opportunity to demonstrate this arises with first-year
students in their first weeks on campus, or with therapists at a meeting
or study day held at a hospital unknown to the participants.

Activity ————————————————————————————

Form three groups of subjects. Each group is given the same
task of finding the way to an unknown location, and returning
to the start.

Group 1 is given a simple map of the route.
Group 2 is given verbal instructions of how to get there.
Group 3 is led through the route, on the outward journey only,
by someone who knows the building.

Note which group returns first (and who does not return!). How important was information about landmarks on the way? Compare the experiences of each group.

The active brain areas in topographical orientation have been investigated by neuro-imaging studies using PET scanning of normal subjects (Maguire *et al.*, 1997, 1998). In the study in 1997, the PET scan was recorded over the time when experienced London taxi drivers were asked to describe the route they would drive from one named location to another around London. In the next study (Maguire *et al.*, 1998), different subjects navigated through a complex virtual reality town. After an initial period of exploration, neuro-imaging was recorded during the performance of various navigational tasks in the virtual town. The results of both these studies showed that activity in the hippocampus in the temporal lobes is strongly associated with navigating between large-scale spatial locations. When the subjects were asked to simply follow arrows through a route in the virtual town, there was greater activity in the right parietal lobe relative to the temporal lobe. In another condition when direct routes were obstructed, so that detours had to be made, the left frontal cortex showed activity.

A navigational system, previously described in animal experiments, has now been proposed in humans (Fig. 4.5). Visual information from the environment reaching the occipital lobes is translated into the spatial components required for navigation by cooperation between the parietal and temporal lobes. The head and the body position in relation to the environment is processed in the right parietal lobe, and an environment-based representation in the hippocampus of the right temporal lobe. The left prefrontal cortex is active when a direct route cannot be followed so that planning and modifying is required (see Chapter 8).

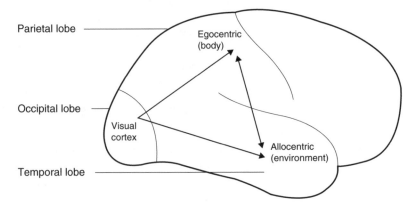

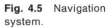

Fig. 4.5 Navigation system.

Summary

(1) The scanning of the features of the space around us demands: an adequate area of intact visual fields; pursuit and saccadic movements of the eyes; and shifts of attention.
(2) Body scheme is the mental representation of the position and the relationship between the parts of the body. Structural, semantic and lexical representations are incorporated into body scheme.
(3) Constructional praxis is the organization of single parts to form one complete item or object. The results produced in drawing figures and constructing block designs have been used to distinguish the spatial and motor components of constructional praxis.
(4) Topographical orientation is a complex ability that involves: the recognition of landmarks and their spatial location with repect to the body and to other landmarks; sequencing of landmarks to form mental representations of routes; and cognitive maps of 'world-centred' knowledge where routes and landmarks are combined.

References

Corbett, A. & Shah, S. (1996) Body scheme disorders following stroke. *British Journal of Occupational Therapy* **59**, 325–9.

Maguire, E. A., Frackowiak, R. S. J. & Frith, C. D. (1997) Recalling routes around London: activation of the right hippocampus in taxi drivers. *Journal of Neuroscience* **17**, 7103–10.

Maguire, E. A., Burgess, N., Donnett, J. G., Frackowiak, R. S. J., Frith, C. D. & O'Keefe, J. (1998) Knowing where and getting there: a human navigation network. *Science* **280**, 921–4.

Sirigu, A., Grafman, J., Bressler, K. & Sunderland, T. (1991) Multiple representations contribute to body knowledge processing: evidence from a case of autopagnosia. *Brain* **114**, 629–42.

Warrington, E. K., James, M. & Kinsbourne, M. (1966) Drawing disability in relation to laterality of cerebral lesion. *Brain* **89**, 53–82.

Chapter 5   Attention

The word 'attention' is part of our everyday vocabulary. We ask others to 'pay attention', or we try to 'catch' the attention of a group. We say we are 'absent minded' when our attention wanders. These examples illustrate how familiar we think we are with attention as part of our actions and behaviour. However, we are unaware of most of the attention processing that forms part of all cognitive functions.

The function of attention is initially to direct the basic perceptual processing of all the modalities of the sensory input from the environment. Attention selects which sensory stimuli are relevant at the time, while irrelevant stimuli are ignored. Further processing in other cognitive systems is then facilitated; for example in memory, both the registration of items and their subsequent retrieval require attention.

We do not perceive everything that is going on in the environment. When we play back an audio recording of a seminar or a meeting, we hear all the sounds that we were not aware of at the time. The brain, on the other hand, orients attention to salient features in the environment, selecting what to listen to and what to look at from moment to moment. Selection also involves shifting attention to a different stimulus. When there are several conversations going on at the same time, we can focus our attention on one of them. However, we may also be monitoring other conversations, especially if our own name is mentioned (Fig. 5.1).

In task performance, habitual well-practised activities involve a low-level attention. Arousal, alertness and vigilance are terms used to describe the attention which is basic to all the activities we perform on 'auto pilot'. However, higher levels of attention processing are required if the same activities are performed in a noisy room or in an unfamiliar environment. This is an important consideration if patients are assessed in the OT department kitchen.

Dividing attention between two or more tasks can be done with varying success, depending on the sensory modalities involved in each and the limitations of the brain's attention capacity. Many students listen to music while they study, keyboard operators have meaningful conversations with colleagues whilst typing, parents perform household tasks and answer the questions of children. Shifts of attention are

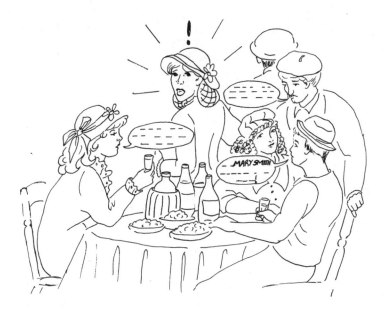

Fig. 5.1 The 'cocktail party phenomenon'.

important for flexibility in behaviour and action. When the telephone rings we make a global shift of attention from the current task in hand to a new goal.

Studies using neuro-imaging have identified brain areas which are active during attention processing. Anatomically distinct areas have been identified for an alerting system and an orienting system with interaction between them for the control of attention processing (Posner & Peterson, 1990).

In neuropsychology, explanations of a syndrome known as unilateral neglect have included an attentional deficit as a primary or secondary cause. The incidence of neglect, usually in right hemisphere lesion, has suggested differences in attention processing between the two sides of the brain.

Many different types of attention have been defined in order to separate the different aspects of attentional behaviour. In this chapter, the components of everyday attention will be divided into three types: sustained, selective and divided attention. In the second part of the chapter, the attentional and related theories which account for the phenomenon of unilateral neglect will be considered.

Components of everyday attention

The type of attention that is the 'base line' for all information processing is sustained attention which includes arousal and alertness.

The type that directs attention to particular features of the environment is known as selective attention. This orients to the relevant sensory input while ignoring others. The ability to do more than one thing at a time depends on divided attention between each of the tasks.

Sustained attention

Arousal has a physiological basis in the activity of the reticular formation in the brain stem. Variations in tonic arousal coincide with diurnal rhythms and also with changes in body temperature or the digestion of food. Faster changes in arousal occur in response to external stimuli, particularly if they are threatening or a quick response is demanded. There are optimum levels of arousal for different activities. For example, tasks which use very fine motor control or have important decision-making components require moderate levels of arousal, rather than the very high arousal which leads to stress.

Alertness is the term used to describe the transition from a wakeful to a 'prepared for action' state when we respond to stimuli at a faster rate. The term 'vigilance' is sometimes used for alertness that is maintained over a period of time in order to detect any change in the environment. A continuous high level of alertness has been called vigilance, and in some cognitive tests the term is used for the minimum time a person can maintain mental alertness.

These endogenous or internal attention mechanisms, including arousal and alertness, can be collectively called sustained attention. All activities demand a level of sustained attention over the time taken to complete them. The maximum length of time that an individual can sustain attention is often called attention span.

Examples of sustained attention are: motorway driving; watching a young child playing alone; observing a patient in occupational therapy. All these tasks require people to maintain sustained attention for long periods of time in order to detect any change which requires action. The driver on the motorway has to be prepared for warning signs of lane closure, or encountering a slow vehicle ahead that must be overtaken.

Selective attention

Selective attention processing involves orienting to the relevant sensory input and inhibiting irrelevant stimuli. Orienting includes sensory discrimination (visual or auditory), and spatial processing. Orienting to a spatial location may include overt movement of the head and eyes towards the point of interest. At other times, covert orienting occurs (without eye movements) when the selected information lies within the current visual fields. The ability to disengage from one selected item, move and engage attention on another source of information is known as attention shifting. The primary cause of loss of attention shifting may be the inability to disengage from the current selected item (see page 52).

Selective attention is important in activities that require a conscious focus of attention, for example reading a newspaper in a room with other people talking. In routine activities, on the other hand, attention is maintained automatically until there is a change in the environment and attention must be shifted to a new input. An example of this is driving to visit a friend after work, on a route that overlaps with the usual route home. There will be a tendency to end up at your own home unintentionally.

Divided attention

Sometimes we want to be engaged in two different things at the same time and this involves divided attention. For example, experienced drivers can have a conversation with a passenger on a journey; some people can knit and watch TV at the same time.

Spelke *et al.* (1976) gave two students the difficult dual task of reading a short story for comprehension at the same time as they wrote down words dictated to them. At first, their speed of reading was slow, and their handwriting was poor. After six weeks of training for five hours a week, they were able to read with speed and understanding, at the same time as writing to dictation.

Dual-task experiments of this kind demonstrate remarkable ability to divide attention between two tasks. When both tasks have high processing demands, new strategies for performing each task may develop, so that there is less interference between them. There is less interference between two tasks that use different sensory modalities; for example, listening to the radio whilst writing is easier than listening to the radio at the same time as holding a conversation.

You can assess your own ability to do more than one thing at a time as follows:

Activity _____

(1) Perform at the same time: a verbal and a visual task; and then two verbal tasks. An example is: recite a poem or rhyme known by heart while (a) matching shapes or objects, and (b) reading a newspaper article. Which is easier?

(2) Watch your favourite soap or sitcom on the TV with a friend. At the same time, copy out your notes from a lecture that day. At the end of the programme, recall the details of what happened in the TV programme to your friend, and ask him/her to question you on the content of the lecture.

Table 5.1 gives a summary of three components of attention:

Table 5.1   The components of attention.

Sustained attention	Endogenous
Arousal, alertness, vigilance	Maintained over time
Selective attention	Shifts of attention
Orienting to selected items	Disengage, move and engage
Divided attention	Two or more tasks

Models of attention

Models that identify where selection occurs in the serial stages of perceptual and semantic processing were developed from studies of how people process two different auditory messages presented at the same time. These studies raised a debate about whether the unattended message is processed before or after the semantic level. There was no evidence of long-term retention of the unattended information, but this could be explained by decay in short-term memory.

An alternative approach, based on the interaction of all the levels of attention processing, produced capacity models of attention. Kahneman (1973) proposed that a central processor of limited capacity allocates attention in parallel to current activities (Fig. 5.2). Problems occur when the demands of the performance of the task(s) exceed the attention capacity.

The demands on attentional capacity vary in several ways:

(1) *Mental effort.* Tasks that involve high mental effort demand a large share of the total attention capacity.
(2) *Skill.* The acquisition of skill at a task, as a result of practice, reduces the attention demands, so that more is available to attend to other tasks.
(3) *Motivation and arousal* increase the total capacity available for allocation.

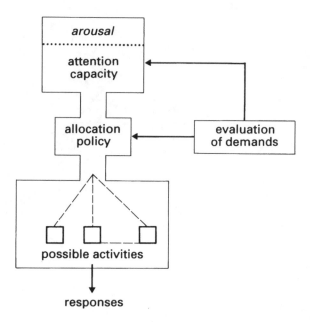

Fig. 5.2 Capacity model of attention (simplified from Kahneman, 1973).

Attention capacity may be reduced after brain damage. Tasks that require high mental effort become too difficult, while tasks that were well learned and familiar now require more attention. General arousal may be reduced so that performance is slow, and concentration is required in all activities. On the other hand, high levels of arousal induce stress and interfere with the performance of complex tasks.

Evidence from PET scan studies confirms that the different types of attention processing are not centred on one brain area alone (Posner *et al.*, 1988). A model of attention proposed by Posner & Peterson (1990) described an anterior alerting and a posterior orienting system which are interrelated:

- *Alerting and vigilance system* located in the prefrontal and anterior cingulate cortex. These areas receives projections from the thalamus and from the arousal system of the brain stem reticular formation (Fig. 5.3a).
- *Orienting system* located in the inferior parietal lobe and superior temporal gyrus (Fig. 5.3b).

The function of the alerting and vigilance system is to prepare the brain for the processing of high-priority signals. The orienting system has a function in both orienting to these signals and also moving attention to a new location when the priority changes.

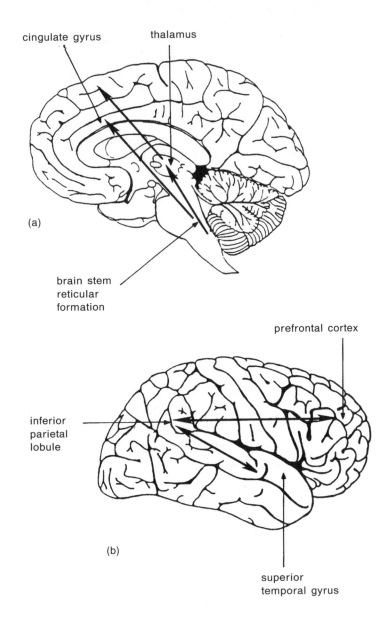

Fig. 5.3 The attentional system: (a) medial view of the right side of the brain seen in sagittal section; (b) side view of the right hemisphere.

Attention in unilateral neglect

Unilateral neglect is a condition which occurs most commonly in patients with lesions in the right parietal lobe. Stimuli on one side of space, usually the left, are ignored. The primary or secondary cause of this phenomenon is an attentional deficit.

The right and left hemispheres each orient attention to cues in the contralateral space (Heilman & Valenstein, 1993) (Fig. 5.4). When the

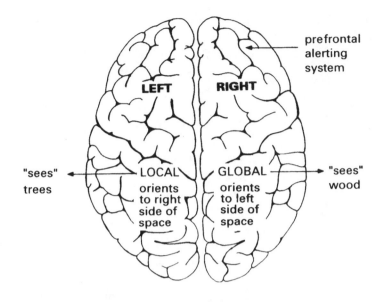

Fig. 5.4 Lateralization of attention processing.

right side is damaged, there is an imbalance in orienting. Attention is always directed to the right, mediated by the left hemisphere, and the left side of space is neglected.

A difference in attentional processing between the right and left parietal lobes has also been shown in relation to the global and local features of the environment. The right parietal lobe directs attention processing to the global features of the environment, processing groups of items simultaneously, while the left parietal lobe emphasizes the local features item by item in a sequential way (Robertson & Lamb, 1991) (Fig. 5.4). Normally a balance exists between these two processes. In neglect, the right hemisphere damage disrupts the global mechanisms of attention so that the patient cannot see the wood for the trees (Warren, 1993).

Heilman and Valenstein also proposed that the right hemisphere is the centre for control of arousal from the reticular formation in the brain stem. In right brain damage, the right hemisphere is under-aroused, and this further biases attention to neglect the left side.

If neglect is a disorder of attention, asking a patient to consciously report the presence of a cue on the neglected side should facilitate the response to information on that side. Studies of the effects of cueing patients to the neglected side in line bisection tests have produced conflicting results. Heilman and Valenstein showed no effect of cueing, while a study by Riddoch & Humphreys (1983) did show that neglect decreased when patients were forced to report a left-sided cue before bisecting the line. The effects of cueing were explored further by Posner *et al.* (1982, 1984). In a series of experiments they investigated the effects of cueing on the response to visual stimuli presented on either side of the midline, in patients with parietal lobe, thalamic or brain stem lesions. One of the findings of the Posner *et al.* experiments showed that neglect patients who are cued to attend to the normal side of space (ipsilateral to the lesion) cannot shift attention to the neglected side to respond to stimuli there. The authors suggested that the primary problem in neglect is the inability to disengage attention from the current focus.

Studies of unilateral neglect support the fractionation of spatial attention into: personal, extrapersonal/reaching, and extrapersonal/ far space (Fig. 4.3). As part of a study of 26 patients with right brain damage, performance on self-care activities in personal space was compared with the use of objects in reaching space (Zoccolatti & Judica, 1991). The results showed that on the neglected side, performance using items in relation to body parts was less impaired than items manipulated in reaching space. A single case study by the same authors showed the opposite effect, i.e. unilateral neglect of personal space, with unimpaired reaching space. Halligan & Marshall (1991) devised a line bisection task in far space. A patient with neglect in reaching space showed no problems when he was asked to bisect a line in far space using a light pointer or (as an experienced darts player) by throwing a dart. These studies suggest that the functional problems experienced by patients with unilateral neglect may be related to different areas of the spatial environment.

Other theories of unilateral neglect

Two alternative explanations of unilateral neglect are a deficit in: spatial perception and the mental representations of one side of space; or, the ability to initiate movement to one side, known as premotor neglect or directional hypokinesia.

The perceptual/representation theory was supported by a classical study by Bisiach & Luzatti (1978). Two patients with left-side neglect were asked to imagine that they were in the Piazza del Duomo in Milan, which was well known to them, standing at each end in turn. When they imagined standing in the square at the end facing the cathedral, the patients described in detail all the buildings on the right side of the square, but the buildings on the left were omitted. When they imagined they were standing at the opposite end of the square on the steps of the cathedral, they described all the buildings that they had neglected before, and omitted the buildings that were now on the left side. Bisiach and Luzatti explained this as an inability to construct a mental representation of the left side of space and the consequent loss of visual imagery on that side.

The intentional theory, also known as premotor neglect or directional hypokinesia, is usually associated with lesions of the right frontal lobe. In the line bisection task, frequently used in research studies of neglect, the patient indicates a position to the right of the midline when asked to mark the midpoint of a line. This could be a difficulty in initiating the movement to make a mark on the left side of the line rather than a loss of either attention or representation of the contralateral space.

The attentional and spatial representation theories may not be distinct since attention is required for spatial processing (Parkin, 1996). Also body scheme disorders may affect the initiation of movements to the opposite side of space. Unilateral neglect has a significant effect on function and the clinical features are varied, both in the detail of the symptoms and in the prognosis. At the present time, there is no single theoretical account of the neglect syndrome (Hartman-Maeir & Katz, 1995).

Summary

(1) Attention processing can be divided into: (a) sustained, which is endogenous and includes arousal, alertness and vigilance; (b) selective, an orienting system involved in focusing and shifting of attention; and (c) divided, which allows two or more tasks to be performed at once.

(2) In a changing environment covert shifts of attention occur, without eye movement, when attention is disengaged from the current focus to move and to engage on a different high-priority stimulus.

(3) The ability to divide attention between tasks depends on the sensory modalities of the input, the nature of the response output, and the amount of practice. Capacity models of attention suggest that problems occur when the allocation of attention to different tasks exceeds the resources available.

(4) The attention system can be divided into: an anterior alerting system in the frontal lobes which receives projections from the thalamus and brain stem reticular formation; and a posterior orienting system in the parietal lobes.

(5) Studies of patients with unilateral neglect support an attentional deficit as the primary or secondary cause. Other explanations include an inability to: form a mental spatial representation; or initiate movement, in the side of space contralateral to the lesion.

References

Bisiach, E. & Luzatti, C. (1978) Unilateral neglect of representational space. *Cortex* **14**, 129–33.

Halligan, P. W. & Marshall, J. C. (1991) Left neglect for near but not far space in man. *Nature* **350**, 498–500.

Hartman-Maeir, A. & Katz, N. (1995) Validity of the Behavioural Inattention Test (BIT); relationships with functional tasks. *American Journal of Occupational Therapy* **49**, 507–16.

Heilman, K. M. & Valenstein, E. (1993) *Clinical Neuropsychology*. New York: Oxford University Press.

Kahneman, D. (1973) *Attention and Effort*. New Jersey: Prentice-Hall.

Parkin, A. J. (1996) Neglect. In *Explorations in Cognitive Neuropsychology*. Oxford: Blackwell Publishers.

Posner, M. I., Cohen, Y., Rafal, R. D. (1982) Neural system control of spatial orienting. *Philosophical Transactions of the Royal Society of London, B* **298**, 187–98.

Posner, M. I., Walker, J. A., Friedrich, F. J. & Rafal, R. D. (1984) Effects of parietal injury on covert orienting of visual attention. *Journal of Neuroscience* **4**, 1863–74.

Posner, M. I., Peterson, S. E., Fox, P. T. & Raichle, M. E. (1988) Localization of cognitive processes in the human brain. *Science* **240**, 1627–31.

Posner, M. I. & Peterson, S. E. (1990) The attentional system of the human brain. *Annual Review of Neuroscience* **13**, 25–42.

Riddoch, M. J. & Humphreys, G. W. (1983) The effect of cueing on unilateral neglect. *Neuropsychologica* **21**, 589–99.

Robertson, L. C. & Lamb, M. R. (1991) Neuropsychological contributions to theories of part/whole organization. *Cognitive Psychology* **23**, 299–330.

Spelke, E. S., Hirst, W. C. & Neisser, U. (1976) Skills of divided attention. *Cognition* **4**, 215–30.

Warren, M. (1993) A hierarchical model for evaluation and treatment of visual perceptual dysfunction. *American Journal of Occupational Therapy* **47**(1), 42–53.

Zoccolatti, P. & Judica, A. (1991) Functional evaluation of hemineglect by means of a semi-structured scale. *Neuropsychological Rehabilitation* **1**, 33–44.

Further reading

Eysenck, M. W. & Keane, M. T. (1990) Attention and performance limitations. In *Cognitive Psychology: A Student's Handbook*, pp. 97–132. London: Lawrence Erlbaum.

Hampson, P. J. & Morris, P. E. (1996) Attention. In *Understanding Cognition*, pp. 111–28. Oxford: Blackwell Publishers.

Chapter 6   Memory

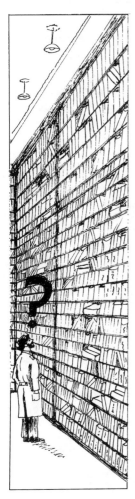

Memory is our ability to keep things in mind, and to recall them sometime in the future. We try to recall names, dates, shopping lists, and the details of journeys we have made, to test our own memory. But everyday memory is also about cooking a meal this evening, or meeting a friend next week at the right time and place. Some aspects of memory are involved in almost everything we do, and the way we use it depends on our own lifestyle and experience.

Memory is often compared with systems that organize and store large amounts of information. A library of books is a static store of information that has been organized in a particular way, but retrieval is slow (Fig. 6.1). Computer systems for information storage do have rapid retrieval, but they are dependent on continual update of the material if they are to remain useful. Memory is a dynamic system that is developed and modified over time, and it is unlikely that access is only available at one location in the brain.

For a long time, investigations of memory in psychology were laboratory based, where conditions for the presentation of the items to be remembered, and their subsequent recall, could be carefully controlled and varied in a predetermined way. It is the results of such rigorous explorations of memory, using lists of digits, letters or words, that led to theories describing the mental processing involved in memory. The importance of attention and perception in memory has been demonstrated. Models of the organization of the stored information into subsystems have been described, together with computer models of how the components may interact in different cognitive abilities.

From the 1970s onwards, some investigations of memory have used material that is related to everyday experiences. Another development has been the exploration of prospective memory for future plans and actions. The most significant effect on the ability to function independently may be the loss of prospective memory for routine activites.

Some impairment of memory occurs in most patients with brain damage. Patients with memory deficits do have residual memory skills and global amnesia is very rare. The prospects for rehabilitation largely depend on the identification of spared memory.

Fig. 6.1 Information storage and retrieval.

Memory can be broadly divided into three systems:

(1) *Sensory memory* is the brief processing of information received by the sense organs that lasts only a few milliseconds before passing on to short-term memory. Sensory memory is modality specific. Visual (iconic) and auditory (echoic) sensory memory have been studied extensively in psychology, but so far there have been few studies of tactile, olfactory and proprioceptive sensory memory.

(2) *Short-term memory* holds information from the sensory memory for several seconds before it is either transferred to long-term memory, or lost due to interference from new items coming in. The original description of a short-term store has been developed into a working memory system where there is rehearsal of items and some active processing for meaning.

(3) *Long-term memory* retains information for periods of time from a few minutes to many years. Forgetting in long-term memory may be due to decay over time, or perhaps the memory remains stored but cannot be retrieved.

Short-term/working memory

The evidence for a short-term memory system is based on the results of free recall of a list of numbers, letters or words.

Activity ———————————————————————

Make a list of 15 words. Choose concrete nouns rather than abstract words or adjectives.

Read the list to a group of colleagues at about one word per second. Then ask them to write down the words in the list that they recall. Check the position in the list of each word recalled by each person.

Repeat with another list, and this time give the group a short exercise in mental arithmetic to do before writing down the words they remember. Again check each recalled word for its position in the list.

The words most frequently recalled will be those at the end of the list. This is known as the recency effect. When the recall was delayed, and the mental arithmetic task was added before recall, the recency effect disappeared.

The recency effect, explored in controlled laboratory conditions, gave support to the presence of a limited-capacity short-term memory system which holds the last few items, usually around seven. The early items in the list (primacy effect) show no change when recall was delayed by another task because they have already entered long-term memory.

Further evidence of a separate short-term memory system is the selective impairment of short-term memory which has been reported in some patients with cerebral damage (Basso *et al.*, 1982).

The exploration of the functions of short-term memory by Baddeley and Hitch in the 1970s led to the development of the working memory system which was later tested and revised. Working memory has several components which select and manipulate verbal, visual and spatial information over several seconds before passing on to long-term memory and also to other cognitive systems.

There are three main components of working memory: a central executive; a phonological loop; and a visuospatial sketchpad (Fig. 6.2).

The *central executive* controls the processing in the other components of working memory by the allocation of attention to each one. The central executive is particularly important when the cognitive demands of a task are high, for example listening to a conversation while reading the newspaper.

The *phonological loop* stores speech-based information in a phonological store (inner ear), and verbally rehearses it in the same order (inner voice). The verbal rehearsal, known as the articulatory system, is repeated in the same order, like an audiotape that is replayed for about two seconds before it decays or passes on into long-term memory. In speaking and reading, several words are held long enough make sense of the words that follow. Words can enter the phonological store directly from the ear, from rehearsal of written or spoken words, and from long-term memory for names of objects or people.

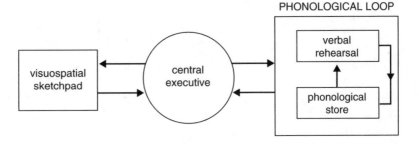

Fig. 6.2 Working memory model.

The *visuospatial sketchpad* stores visual and spatial information entering from the eye over a few seconds in time. This 'inner eye' component of working memory holds both spatial information and visual images that cannot be rehearsed verbally, such as size, shape, colour and distance. It can also be used to inspect and manipulate visual images entering from the eyes or from long-term memory. In finding our way around, 'snapshots' of visual and spatial information are held for a short time to allow us to recognize landmarks.

The working memory model offers an account of how the abundance of sensory information continually entering the brain is processed over a brief period of time before passing on to the other components of the perceptual and cognitive systems. The central executive component of working memory has been least explored. It may be part of the supervisory attention system in the frontal lobes (see Chapter 8). A comprehensive account of working memory can be found in Cohen *et al.* (1993).

Long-term memory

The long-term memory system has unlimited capacity and processes a large variety of information. Items from working memory enter long-term memory where they are processed for meaning and context. Stored memories in long-term memory are retrieved into working memory before the relevant response is activated, for example speech or action. Figure 6.3 shows how the three main memory systems interact.

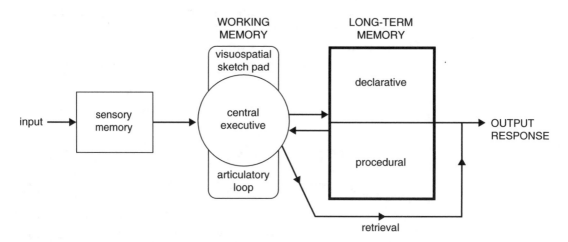

Fig. 6.3 The three memory systems.

Long-term memory has been separated into different subsystems which process and store particular kinds of information. The identification of specific types of memory deficit can help to predict functional problems and guide the choice of aids for a memory-impaired person. However, debate continues in cognitive psychology about the divisions in long-term memory and how they interact (Hampson & Morris, 1996).

Procedural memory – how?

Procedural memory is the subsystem related to the performance of learned skilled activity. All the motor and language skills that we have learnt are part of procedural memory. We remember how to swim, to ride a bicycle, to drive a golf ball accurately, but we cannot explain in detail how to do it. We can speak our first language without knowing the complicated rules of grammar that are associated with it. Procedural memory is implicit and cannot be inspected consciously. It may be called 'knowing how'.

The knowledge of learned motor skills stored in procedural memory is linked to the specific conditions for the actions involved. Activation of the correct procedure depends on matching of the input conditions from working memory, and from decision-making. Skilled actions become more automatic with practice. One reason for this may be that repetition of the particular condition/action pair in procedural memory leads to easier and faster activation.

Procedural memory is spared in most patients with memory loss, so that motor skills well learned before cerebral damage are retained. This has important implications for the return to work and for the continuation of leisure pursuits in memory-impaired individuals. Some patients with language impairment retain their first language when a previously fluent second language is lost.

Declarative memory – what?

Declarative memory is the recollection of knowledge of people, objects, places and events, and that certain facts are true or false. It can be called 'knowing what'. When we are asked a concrete question, for example 'Where were you born?', we consciously inspect declarative memory to recall the name of the place.

Declarative memory has been divided into: semantic memory which is general knowledge of facts; and episodic memory which constitutes memories linked to a time and place. Semantic memory is knowing that Rome is the capital of Italy and bananas are yellow. Episodic memory is a record of particular events, for example knowing where you spent a holiday last year, or the first trip you made by plane.

The distinction between semantic and episodic is blurred and the two types interact in everyday memory. Knowledge that began as episodic becomes generalized into semantic memory over time. Learning to use a microcomputer may at first be associated with a particular model in a college laboratory (episodic). After a time, the operation of a computer becomes part of our general knowledge of the world, which is semantic memory.

Autobiographical memory is another component of declarative memory. Episodic and autobiographical both have a context in time and space, but autobiographical memory is linked to specific life events which have significance for the individual. These life events are important for knowledge of ourselves, family and friends together with our collective experiences of the past. Loss of autobiographical memory reduces self-esteem and can be distressing for the individual.

Implicit memory is the evidence of stored knowledge without awareness. Studies of amnesic patients have shown that patients perform badly on tests of explicit recall but they can learn new skills. The classic example of implicit memory is from Clarapede in 1911 who hid a pin in his hand before shaking hands with one of his amnesic patients. She was subsequently reluctant to shake hands with him but she could not say why. Some amnesic patients show improvement in the performance of leisure tasks, for example jigsaws, without awareness of the change. More research is needed into the ways in which implicit memory in patients with memory deficits can be exploited in the performance of tasks.

Prospective memory – when?

Prospective memory is remembering what to do and when to do it. It is explicit memory which requires attention processing.

Laboratory studies of memory have been concerned with retrospective memory, but a large part of everyday memory is prospective. Stored plans for action need to be activated in the future, on the right day at the right time. The time may be specific (go to a meeting at 2 o'clock), or within a period of time (put the plants in the garden when it stops raining). Prospective memory involves the ability to monitor time and to keep track of ongoing actions. It may also include decisions about the priority of competing plans, for example 'have lunch' or 'complete report writing'. Prospective memory may be described as remembering 'when'.

Prospective memory has some elements of retrospective memory. Remembering to take tablets at intervals in the day includes the recall of how many and the colour of each type.

Everyday routine tasks are mostly automatic and they are performed with minimal demands on prospective memory. In non-routine actions, which have to be remembered once in a while, prospective memory is needed to activate the plan at the right time. Sometimes there is an external cue to activate the plan, for example a letter-box on the way home prompts you to post a letter. In the absence of a cue, the attention demands in working memory may affect the success or failure of prospective memory. We forget to make an important phone call when there are many demands on our attention.

Investigations of prospective memory have included self-rating questionnaires which ask people to record when omissions occurred in their plans for the day. However, the reliability of self-rating depends on the subject's general awareness. Other studies have set subjects specific tasks, such as making a phone call at a particular time or posting a letter on a specific day, with variations in the number of actions to be remembered and the time interval between giving the instruction and the execution of the action. The results of these studies are summarized in Harris (1984).

Prospective memory involves the interaction of memory with other cognitive systems. The executive functions operate on stored plans for action in flexible problem-solving (see Chapter 8).

Summary of long-term memory

Memory has been described in terms of its structure and organization into subsystems. Some of these divisions overlap, for example semantic and episodic memory, and evidence of a distinction between them is weak. The study of people with memory deficits in neuropsychology does provide evidence of selective impairment of subsystems in long-term memory. A summary of long-term memory as described in this section is given in Fig. 6.4.

Registration, retention and retrieval

The studies of memory that are based on the processes that operate in the long-term memory system have identified three stages: registration or coding at the time of learning; retention or storage over time; retrieval of information when it is required. These stages can be remembered as the three Rs.

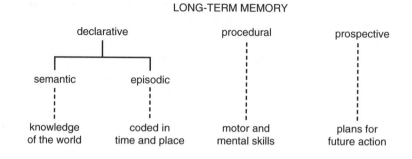

Fig. 6.4 Summary of the structure of long-term memory.

Registration has been explored by manipulating the features and the context of the infomation that is learnt, and testing the subsequent recall to see what factors are most important. Information that is elaborated and processed with meaning at the time of registration increases the likelihood of later retrieval. We are more likely to remember someone's name if we also learn other personal details about family and where he or she lives than if we only register physical appearance. Some of the strategies we use to improve memory use elaboration and association; for example, retracing our steps to remember where we put something, or associating the name of a person with visual imagery of his or her unique features.

Retention is a dynamic process. Stored knowlege is modified and updated by new information entering from working memory over time. Once an item has been registered in memory, subsequent forgetting could be the result of decay over time, or it could be due to interference by later learning. Recall of an event depends on the number of similar events that have occurred, rather than the time that has elapsed, suggesting that interference has an effect. The loss of neurotransmitters has been linked to poor registration and storage in memory, for example in Alzheimer's and Korsakoff's diseases (Kopelman, 1986). More research into the effect of drugs that stimulate the production of these transmitters may confirm this.

Retrieval involves active cognitive processing. Recall is a search process followed by a decision process, while recognition only involves the decision process, so that recognition is easier than recall.

Retrieval is affected by the context, and items are more likely to be retrieved in the same environment as they were learnt. New learning in the hospital OT department may not generalize to the home environment.

External cueing is an important aid to retrieval of items or events from memory. Recall of the name of a person is improved if it is cued by the first letter or other information about the person. Recognition of the person from a group of names or photographs will assist successful retrieval.

We are all familiar with the 'tip of the tongue phenomenon' when we know an item is in memory but we cannot retrieve it. One explanation is that the current processing does not match the stored information and fails to cue the memory. Some implicit retrieval may occur which is activated at a later time and recall is achieved.

Mood also affects retrieval. Experimental studies of the effects of drugs have shown that learning in the altered state can be recalled better in the same state. Depressed patients easily recall memories of sad events and this can add to their depression (Teasdale, 1983).

Schema theory

The organization of the complex knowledge associated with actions and events has posed a question for many studies in cognitive psychology. We retrieve the same generic knowledge in many different situations, and we experience the same events in different contexts. Schema theory proposes that packets of stored knowledge relating to one situation are organized as a schema (plural: schemas or schemata). The knowledge contained in a schema can be simple or complex, ranging from an object to knowledge of the world. A complex schema related to an event has been called a script. Schemas grow with experience and they are transformed into a typical form which interprets the incoming information to fit with prior expectations.

A possible framework of a schema for 'shopping' is given in Fig. 6.5, based on Cohen *et al.* (1993), Part I section 3. The schema specifies the knowledge that is common to all shopping: place, equipment, people and actions, known as the slots. Each slot contains the concepts or actions related to it, with default values if information is not available. The optional values are acquired from particular episodes of shopping.

Stored schemas interpret the input from the environment to make the best fit by top-down perceptual processing. This was illustrated in an experiment by Brewer & Treyens (1981) who asked 30 subjects to spend 35 seconds in a room that looked like an office. Objects were present in the room that were: relevant to an office; not appropriate for an office (e.g. a piece of bark); or in unusual places, for example a notepad on a chair rather than a desk. After leaving the room, they were unexpectedly asked to recall the objects in the room. Recall

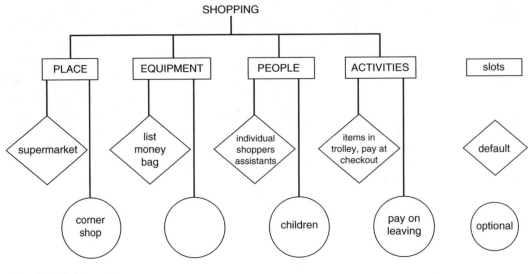

Fig. 6.5 Schema theory.

errors were greatest for items that did not fit into a prototypical office schema, and some subjects recalled items likely to be in an office that were not present.

Schema theory began in the 1930s when Bartlett presented English subjects with a North American folk tale which was completely unfamiliar to Western culture. When they were later asked to recall the tale, the accounts were reconstructed to fit the expectations from their own experience. More recent studies of eyewitness testimony have also shown that the recall of an event at a later date can be affected by exposure to new information in the time interval between the event and recall (Loftus, 1975). This confirms that schemas may be modified and updated over time.

Schema theory does not account for all the features of everyday memory and it has been criticized as being too simple. It does provide a framework for the way that complex knowledge, incorporating different types of memory, may be stored in the brain. The schema approach to the organization of action sequences is discussed in Chapter 7, pp. 71–2.

Summary

(1)   Working memory theory is an account of how verbal and visuospatial information from the environment is held for a few

seconds while some active processing for meaning occurs. Verbal (speech-based) is rehearsed in the phonological loop. Attention is allocated between the visual and verbal components by a central executive. Information retrieved from long-term memory is processed in working memory during recall.

(2)   The structure of long-term memory can be divided into three subsystems. (a) Declarative memory for facts and events, that is retrieved by conscious awareness. It can be called 'knowing what'. (b) Procedural memory for learned motor and verbal skills which does not involve conscious access. It can be called 'knowing how'. (c) Prospective memory is a store of plans for future action and behaviour which are usually recalled without external cues. It can be called 'knowing when'.

(3)   Processing in long-term memory includes three stages: registration at the time of learning, which depends on the level of processing, elaboration, and context; retention over time, which may be affected by modification and interference from new memories; and retrieval, which can be achieved with or without awareness, and it is affected by context and mood.

(4)   Schema theory describes how stored knowledge relating to one situation (object, person, action or event) may be organized. Schemas develop as a result of past experience and they guide the selection of current input to meet expectations.

References

Basso, A., Spinnler, H., Vallar, G. & Zanobio, E. (1982) Left hemisphere damage and selective impairment of auditory verbal short-term memory: a case study. *Neuropsychologia* **20**, 263–74.

Brewer, W. F. & Treyens, J. C. (1981) Role of schemata in memory for places. *Cognitive Psychology* **13**, 207–30.

Cohen, G., Kiss, G. & LeVoi, M. (1993) *Memory: Current Issues*. Buckingham: Open University Press.

Hampson, P. J. & Morris, P. E. (1996) Chapter 2 Memory and Chapter 7 Remembering. In *Understanding Cognition*, pp. 17–48 and 153–74. Oxford: Blackwell Publishers.

Harris, J. E. (1984) Remembering to do things in everyday memory. In *Everyday Memory, Actions and Absent Mindedness* (J. E. Harris & P. E. Morris, eds), pp. 71–92. London: Academic Press.

Kopelman, M. D. (1986) The cholinergic neurotransmitter system in human memory and dementia: a review. *Quarterly Journal of Experimental Psychology* **38a**, 535–74.

Loftus, E. F. (1975) Leading questions and the eyewitness report. *Cognitive Psychology* **7**, 560–72.

Teasdale, J. D. (1983) Affect and accessibility. *Philosophical Transactions of the Royal Society of London* **B302**, 403–12.

Further reading

Baddeley, A. D. (1992) *Your Memory: A User's Guide*. London: Penguin Books.
Cohen, G. (1989) *Memory in the Real World*. Hove: Erlbaum.

Chapter 7   Task Performance

In the execution of all movement, the output from the motor centres in the brain activates patterns of activity in the muscles which move the various segments of the body involved. If the movement is part of the performance of a task, objects are manipulated and actions are modified during the task in response to changes in the environment. The sensory system is active to process visual and tactile information from the objects as well as visual and auditory cues from the environment. In task performance there is a goal for the movement and a sequence of actions must be executed in the correct order to reach that goal. Patients who show poor task performance may have motor and/ or sensory deficits which can be identified by the assessment of sensation, muscle tone, motor patterns, reciprocal innervation and balance reactions. Other patients, however, with minimal motor or sensory loss, have difficulties in the execution of object-oriented movement, particularly when the task uses more than one object. These problems originate in the cognitive system.

Information processing models of motor behaviour have been developed from studies of the acquisition of motor skills in normal subjects. In cognitive neuropsychology, single case studies of patients with cerebral damage have identified serial and parallel modules of praxis processing for the execution of gestures and of movements related to object use.

The mental processing for the performance of a task includes many components of cognition. Perceptual input is integrated with recognition processes related to objects and the actions associated with their use. Correct matching between the object and the action must occur at each stage in a sequence of actions. A mismatch, between an object and the action related to it, is seen in performance errors (Fig. 7.1). Attention demands range from the automatic processing in routine automatic tasks, to the controlled processing required for learning a new task in an unfamiliar environment. Working memory selects the relevant environmental cues, and stored procedural knowledge of skilled movement is recalled from long-term memory. The accurate execution of the task by the motor system depends on all these cognitive processes.

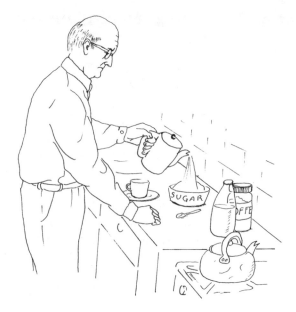

Fig. 7.1 Mismatch of object and action in a sequence with multiple objects.

Programs for action

In the 1970s, psychologists who were interested in the acquisition of motor skills adopted an information processing approach to normal motor behaviour. The term 'motor program' was introduced to describe a stored action memory for a particular movement. The original concept of a motor program was extended into a motor schema which incorporates the perceptual as well as the motor components of movement (Schmidt, 1975). Schema theory, developed in cognitive psychology, proposes that knowledge of the component actions in a daily living task are organized into a family of schemas which are activated in a particular order to reach the goal. The definitions of the terms 'motor program' and 'motor schemas' will now be considered.

The motor program

The early description of the motor program was a set of motor commands that executes movement. The motor program specified not only which muscles are active but also the direction, force and timing of the muscle activity. This can be compared with a computer program which executes a series of functions when the program is activated. One problem with this original definition of a motor program is that it does not account for the execution of a particular movement by different groups of muscles. For example, you can write your signature using different muscle groups.

Activity ─────────────────────────────

Sign your name on a small piece of paper using the fingers and thumb to move the pencil. Then sign your name on a wall-mounted board using the muscles of the shoulder and the elbow. The signature is the same, even though different muscle groups have been used in each case.

The motor program for a simple ballistic movement is programmed before the start. If you press a computer key or throw a piece of paper into a waste basket, once you have started there is no chance of changing the movement. This is known as open loop movement (Fig. 7.2a). Accuracy can be improved in open loop movement so there must be some option for change in the motor program before the start of the action.

Most of our actions take longer, and we do make changes during the progress of the movement in response to feedback. In pouring water from a kettle into a cup, the movement is modified as it proceeds in response to the weight of the kettle (proprioceptive feedback),

(a)
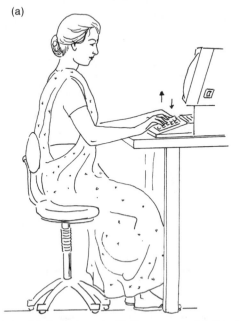

(b)
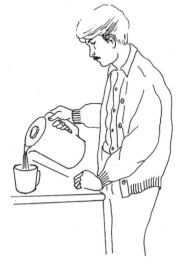

Fig. 7.2 (a) Open loop ballistic movements; (b) closed loop movement with feedback.

and to the level of the water in the cup (visual feedback). This is known as closed loop movement (Fig. 7.2b). A closed loop model developed by Adams (1971) (Fig. 7.3) shows feedback of sensory information from the proprioceptors in the muscles of the moving limbs and from exteroceptors (visual, auditory and tactile). There are now two memory traces for each movement:

- the action memory trace that activates the movement (motor program)
- the perceptual trace which grows as a function of feedback.

The role of feedback in this model is to increase the strength of the perceptual memory trace. In the early stages of learning, when the perceptual trace is weak and poorly defined, intrinsic error correction is poor, and the benefits of verbal prompting and cueing are great. In the later stage of learning, the perceptual trace is strong, and error correction can be based on proprioceptive feedback alone. Adams suggested that the perceptual trace becomes a proprioceptive image, similar to a visual image in memory.

Poor execution of movement after cerebral damage can be explained as the loss of stored motor programs, or of the ability to construct or modify them. Perceptual deficits may reduce the possibility for error correction during the progress of movement. A criticism of the Adams model is the large storage capacity that would be required for the motor programs of the number of movements we make.

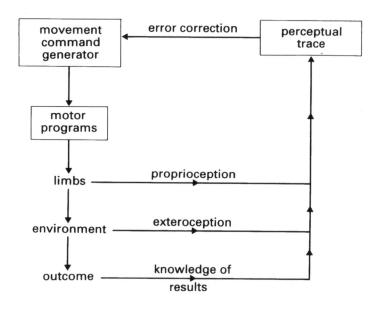

Fig. 7.3 Closed loop model (Adams, 1971).

Action schemas

Schmidt (1975) described a motor (action) schema as a generalized motor program activated for all the movements associated with a common motor pattern. For example, a motor schema for reaching and grasping can be related to a cup on a table, a packet of food in a cupboard, or the hand of a child. The difference between these movement patterns is the direction and extent (force) of the movement, and the constraints of the object being grasped.

Schema theory suggests that a motor schema for a particular movement pattern grows with practice in different situations. This supports the value of variable practice in the early stages of learning. A motor schema for reaching and grasping is strengthened by practice of all the activities that incorporate this movement pattern. The principle of normal movement used widely in physical rehabilitation, which incorporates the facilitation of normal movement patterns in all daily living activities, is supported by schema theory.

Norman (1981) extended the motor schema for a movement pattern to develop a hierarchical model for all the action schemas involved in a routine activity. A high-level or 'parent' schema defines the goal of the action. Low-level or 'child' schemas define the component actions to achieve the goal. A low-level schema can be called a sub-schema. Figure 7.4 outlines the organization of a schema for making a hot drink.

Each high-level schema has a set of triggering conditions for activation. When the wrong high-level schema is triggered, intention errors are made. We experience this goal-switching when we arrive at the supermarket when our intention was to go to the post office.

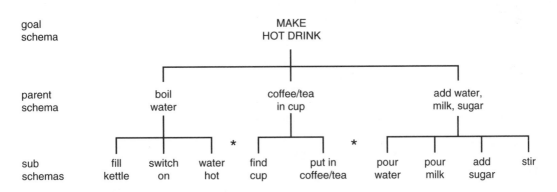

* transition point

Fig. 7.4 Hierarchy of action schemas.

During the progress of complex movements, there are transition points from one subschema to the next and there is option for switching to a different one in response to changes in environmental input. Errors occur frequently at transition points from one subschema to the next. Boiling the kettle is followed by inserting the tea or coffee into a cup. An omission error at this transition point can lead to pouring water into an empty cup with no tea or coffee. Other errors at this point in a sequence may be: repetitions; intrusion of irrelevant actions; and actions made in relation to the wrong object.

Activity

Make a list of action errors you make in different situations; for example, washing and dressing, meal preparation, leaving the house to go to work, driving, or walking to the shops.

Compare your list with others in a group. Are there individual differences? When do action errors occur more frequently?

Similar errors made by normal subjects are seen in patients with cerebral damage, particularly perseveration (repetition of action) at a transition point, when there is inability to move on to the next action subschema in the sequence. This is a common feature of dyspraxia (see Chapter 14).

Models of praxis

The word 'praxis' means movement. The term 'apraxia' is used in neuropsychology to name disorders of the execution of purposeful movement in the absence of sensory loss, muscle weakness, ataxia or incomprehension.

Neuroanatomical model

In 1905, Liepmann was the first to use the term 'apraxia' to describe a movement disorder associated with using tools and objects. Liepmann's patients with apraxia all had left hemisphere lesions and he established the left hemisphere as dominant for movement as well as language. He described a neuroanatomical model of praxis (Fig. 7.5).

More recent studies by Geschwind (1975) and Heilman *et al.* (1982) confirmed that action memories for the movements involved in the use of tools are stored in the parietal lobe contralateral to the dominant hand. In the performance of a task, the left parietal lobe receives visual and spatial perceptual processing of the objects and the environment from both the occipital and the right parietal lobes (see Chapters 3 and 4). The left parietal lobe projects to the left frontal motor areas for the execution of movements of the right upper limb. For skilled movements of the left side of the body, the activity crosses to the motor areas of the right frontal lobe via the corpus callosum (Fig. 7.5).

The motor areas in the frontal lobe include the primary motor cortex on each side that activate the muscles on the opposite side of the body via the corticospinal pathways. Two other motor areas lie anterior to the primary motor cortex: the supplementary motor area (SMA) which receives projections from the parietal lobe; and the premotor area which receives visual perceptual processing from the occipital lobes. Both these areas have projections to the primary motor area.

Physiological studies have shown that during complex movements all the frontal motor areas are active, but the SMA neurones discharge before the neurones in the primary motor area (Brinkman &

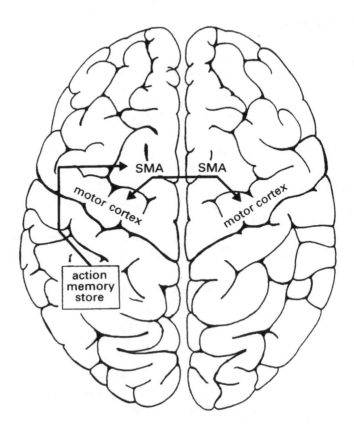

Fig. 7.5 Neuroanatomical model of praxis (SMA – supplementary motor area).

Porter, 1979). This suggests that the SMA translates the time and space memory representation stored in the left parietal lobe into the correct motor pattern for projection to the primary motor cortex. Goldberg (1985) demonstrated activity in the premotor area when the occipital lobes were activated by visual input from the external environment. An analogy proposed by Goldberg is that the premotor and SMA areas cooperate in the control of activity in the primary motor area in the same way that the pilot and the navigator control the flight of an aeroplane.

The neuroanatomical model of praxis outlines a system which integrates:

- the left parietal lobe which stores semantic (conceptual) knowledge of objects and the actions related to their use; with
- the motor areas in the frontal lobes which execute the correct spatial and temporal features of gestures and object-oriented movements.

The outcome of disruption in each of these areas will be considered in Chapter 14.

Information processing model

Studies of praxis in cognitive neuropsychology have identified modules of processing in series and in parallel from auditory (to command) and visual (by imitation) inputs to output in action and naming. To date there have been few studies of the processing of tactile input from objects.

A simplified model of the stages of processing described by Rothi *et al.* (1991) is shown in Fig. 7.6.

- The input stages are modules of visual analysis (perceptual) and auditory analysis (verbal commands).
- The object recognition system includes viewer- and object-centred representations (see Chapter 3).
- The semantic system. Roy & Square (1985) proposed that action semantics includes three kinds of knowledge: object function; actions into which objects can be incorporated; and sequences of action.
- The action output lexicon is stored knowledge of the actions associated with objects. Rothi *et al.* (1991) introduced the term 'action lexicon', proposing similarities with the speech output

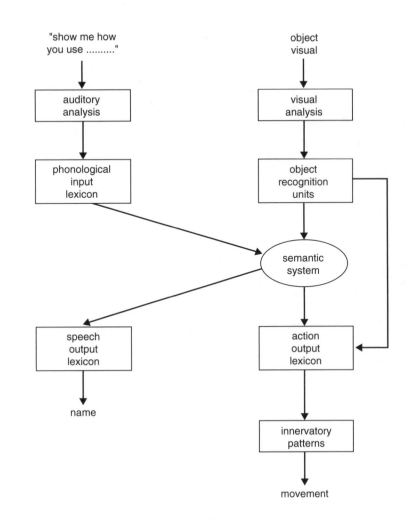

Fig. 7.6 Generation of action from visual and verbal routes (based on Rothi *et al.*, 1991).

lexicon for naming. An example of activation of the action lexicon would be: matching the conditions of a jug filled with water held in the hand with an action schema for tilting and pouring.

- The innervatory patterns for the sequence of actions involved in the movement (Rothi *et al.*, 1991) incorporate information about the position of body parts in relation to each other and to the surfaces of the objects being manipulated.
- The motor system executes the innervatory patterns.

Action generated by command follows the auditory/verbal input shown on the left in Fig. 7.6. Evidence for a dissociation between the auditory/verbal route and the visual/object route to the action system is seen when a patient can use objects he or she cannot name. Some dyspraxic patients with language problems can copy the gestures of object use performed by a therapist using the visual/gestural route from vision to the action semantic system.

The modules in the model can be separated into two parts: the praxis conceptual (semantic) system; and the praxis production system. These two levels have parallels with the two stages of the neuroanatomical account.

Summary

(1) In the complex closed loop movements involved in task performance, action memories are elaborated by feedback of perceptual input from the objects and the environment.

(2) Schema theory applied to task performance suggests that action memories are organized into sets which develop with practice. Task performance then depends on the activation of the appropriate high-level schema to reach the goal. Subschemas are activated in serial order, and action errors frequently occur at transition points from the activation of one subschema to the next in the sequence of actions involved.

(3) Liepmann's neuroanatomical model of praxis linked the performance of skilled purposeful movements to the left hemisphere. Action memories stored in the left parietal lobe project to the motor areas of the left frontal lobe for movements of the right upper limb. Learned movements of the left upper limb are activated via the corpus callosum to the motor areas of the right frontal lobe.

(4) Information processing models of praxis have identified two components: the conceptual (semantic) and the production systems. The conceptual system processes knowledge of: the function of objects; the actions related to object function; and the sequencing of action. The production system processes the output from the conceptual system to specify the time and space relations of movement and activate the motor system for the execution of the movement.

References

Adams, J. A. (1971) A closed loop theory of motor behaviour. In *Motor Control: Issues and Trends* (G. E. Stelmach, ed.). New York: Academic Press.

Brinkman, C. & Porter, R. (1979) Supplementary motor area in the monkey: activity of neurones during performance of a learned motor task. *Neurophysiology* **42**, 681–709.

Geschwind, N. (1975) The apraxias: neural mechanisms of disorders of learned movements. *American Scientist* **63**, 188–95.

Goldberg, G. (1985) Response and projection: a reinterpretation of the pre-motor concept. In *Neuropsychological Studies of Apraxia and Related Disorders* (E. A. Roy, ed.). Amsterdam: Elsevier.

Heilman, K. M., Rothi, L. J. & Valenstein, E. (1982) Two forms of ideomotor apraxia. *Neurology* **32**, 342–6.

Norman, D. A. (1981) Categorization of action slips. *Psychological Review* **88**, 1–15.

Rothi, L. J. G., Ochipa, C. & Heilman, K. M. (1991) A cognitive neuro-psychological model of limb praxis. *Cognitive Neuropsychology* **8**(6), 443–58.

Roy, E. A. & Square, P. A. (1985) Common considerations in the study of limb, verbal and oral apraxia. In *Neuropsychological Studies of Apraxia and Related Disorders* (E. A. Roy, ed.). Amsterdam: Elsevier.

Schmidt, R. A. (1975) A schema theory of discrete motor skill learning. *Psychological Review* **82**, 225–60.

Further reading

Rothi, L. J. G. & Heilman, K. M. (eds) (1997) *Apraxia: The Neuropsychology of Action*. Hove: Psychology Press.

Chapter 8   Executive Functions

All our perceptual and cognitive skills are integrated at a high level by the executive system. This allows us to formulate goals, to set plans, and to organize and monitor tasks. The executive system works out what information is relevant in order to make effective decisions, and develops tactics to deal with changes when they occur.

At home, at work and in leisure time we do everyday tasks automatically. When a new situation arises, however, we have to make decisions about what to do and how to do it (Fig. 8.1). We may be aware of a similar situation in the past and try to remember how we dealt with it. A successful solution will depend on our ability to set a realistic goal, make a plan and keep an eye on how the plan is progressing.

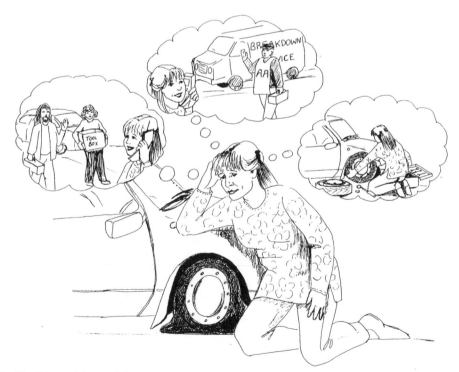

Fig. 8.1 Flexible problem-solving.

The executive functions are the cognitive processes involved in the 'what to do' and 'how to do it' of action and behaviour. They direct and regulate all the other cognitive functions. In order to do this, there must be interaction with self-awareness and insight. Operating on stored procedural knowledge, effective strategies are monitored and modified when the demands change. The output of executive processing interacts with stored schemas for movement and language to activate the response.

The importance of the prefrontal cortex for executive processing has been identified from frontal lobe lesion studies and from recent neuro-imaging in normal subjects. This confirms the location of a high-level component of the attention system which controls non-routine activity.

Some of the terminology in neuropsychology associated with the executive functions appears to overlap with that used in both motor performance and attention. For example, planning, programming, initiation and perseveration are cognitive operations in motor performance (see Chapter 7). When applied to executive functions, these terms are qualitatively different and operate at higher levels of control.

Automatic and controlled processing

It is common experience that well-learned and practised activities become automatic. For a large part of the day we function on 'auto-pilot'. Stored schemas for action and for thought are refined with practice (see Chapter 7). Each schema is triggered by the environment or from the output of other schemas. Entering my room to do word processing in the evening, a schema for switching on the light is activated by the input from the room in darkness and the act of opening the door. Component subschemas are then activated automatically to walk to the word processor, sit down and switch on.

At times, the routine selection of a schema may not be appropriate for the situation. The relative importance of different responses is assessed, the routine schema is inhibited and another schema is selected. The first stage of your journey home from work may be triggered by locking the office door which activates the schema for walking to the station, the bus stop, or the car. This all occurs automatically unless you came by car and have to search for where you left it that morning. A different schema must be activated if you are going to a meeting after work, and this requires inhibition of the 'going home' schema after locking the door. If a patient is waiting for you when you lock the door, your response now demands decision-making and active control of future action.

The difference between automatic and controlled processing was studied by Shiffrin & Schneider (1977) using laboratory-based visual tasks. In these experiments, it was shown that:

- automatic processes are fast, do not require attention, but they are difficult to modify;
- controlled processes are relatively slow, demand attention, but they are flexible when circumstances change.

These laboratory studies distinguished two types of processing that occur in tasks that involved visual attention, but did not explain how processing changes from controlled to automatic as a result of practice.

Routine and non-routine tasks

The executive functions are concerned with the overall organization of cognition and action. Deficits in this system can lead to problems in carrying out any tasks that require initiation, planning and organizing, or may even result in the complete avoidance of any non-routine activity.

A model was developed by Norman and Shallice (Shallice, 1982) to predict the difference between the performance of routine and non-routine tasks. Drawing on the approach of computer modelling in cognitive science, the model gives a useful account of our responses to relevant cues, ignoring others that are irrelevant, and to the monitoring of ongoing behaviour.

In the model (Fig. 8.2) the perceptual input from the environment is processed in a trigger database which in turn accesses the stored schemas for routine activities. Evidence from studies of action errors (Norman, 1981) suggests that conflict can occur in schema selection when the same environmental trigger can activate different schemas. In the 'leave work' example previously mentioned, there was conflict between the schema for walking to the car, and walking to the meeting room. The selection of the appropriate schema, and the inhibition of all conflicting schemas, is called contention scheduling. This determines the priority of one set of actions over others. Habitual behaviour is adjusted to meet the demands of the situation. Failure in

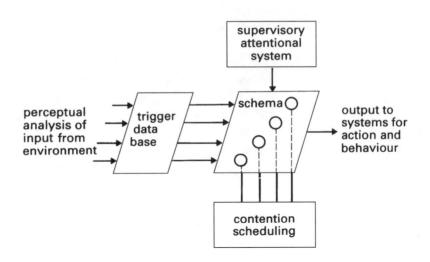

Fig. 8.2 Model of attention control in executive functions (based on Shallice, 1982).

contention scheduling results in action errors and you may find yourself at the bus stop instead of the meeting room.

Situations do arise when the routine selection of action by contention scheduling may be inappropriate, and actions are required that involve decision-making. An example is driving to a friend's house one day instead of taking a habitual route home from work. In the Norman and Shallice model, the selection of the schema for willed actions is controlled by a supervisory activation system (SAS), also known as a supervisory attention system. This system, which allows for decision-making to achieve a novel goal, can be impaired independently from the attentional processing in routine tasks (Shallice, 1982).

The Norman and Shallice model identifies three different levels of function:

(1) automatic processing, based on schema selection, for habitual action and thought
(2) contention scheduling to resolve conflict in schema selection
(3) controlled processing by a supervisory activation system for flexible responses to new situations.

Contention scheduling is partially automatic with more awareness than fully automatic processing.

There is neuropsychological evidence that the supervisory activation system is located in the frontal lobes. This will be considered in the next section.

The frontal lobes

For more than a century, neurologists observing patients with frontal lobe damage have commented on their inability to: make decisions; initiate action or thought; or reach short- and long-term goals. Luria (1966) described these features as frontal lobe syndrome, which is now known as dysexecutive syndrome (DES). The effects of frontal lobe damage are varied, especially when other brain areas are involved, but a common theme is the disorganization of activity which may be expressed across memory, language, movement or problem-solving with failure to achieve known goals (Duncan, 1986). Patients with frontal lobe lesion may achieve normal levels in the assessment of routine task performance, but they are unable to organize their own life. Functional imaging studies (Frith *et al.*, 1991; Passingham, 1996) have demonstrated activity in the prefrontal and anterior cingulate cortex of the frontal lobe (Fig. 5.3) when normal subjects were asked to generate movements at will. Activity was not present in the same frontal areas when the subjects copied the experimenter's finger movements, or practised a sequence of hand movements for one hour so that the actions had become automatic. These PET scan studies have confirmed that actions requiring decision-making involve the prefrontal area while familiar or practised actions do not.

Flexible problem-solving

In problem-solving, the executive functions interact with other cognitive skills, for example attention, memory and planning. Sustained attention is basic to all problem-solving activity, and mental flexibility depends on attention-switching. Processing in memory includes contention scheduling which operates on stored schemas in retrospective memory. Also stored plans in prospective memory execute ongoing actions at the appropriate time.

Effective planning and organization involves the activation of strategies or routines that select and guide the processing of information from the environment. During the progress of a task, conditions may change and different strategies are selected until the goal is reached.

If we take an example of a flat tyre on a car (Fig. 8.1), the goal is to acquire a functional wheel and tyre. This will involve several stages:

- Stage 1   Identify the problem and the solution.
- Stage 2   Formulate a plan and organize actions. The plan may be to change the tyre yourself, or to call for help from a friend or from a breakdown service.

- Stage 3   Monitor the activity and correct it if the tyre remains flat.
- Stage 4   If the goal is not reached, modify the plan and monitor it until the tyre is inflated.

The choice of processing strategies requires the ability to estimate both task difficulty and the time needed to complete the task. In the example of the flat tyre, the most effective strategy may be to leave the car and go home by bus.

A Multiple Errands Task was devised by Shallice & Burgess (1991) to investigate problem-solving ability. Three patients with frontal lobe lesions and nine control subjects were given instructions to complete eight tasks in a shopping precinct. Six of the tasks were related to shopping (for example, buy a brown loaf). The seventh task required the person to be in a specific place 15 minutes after starting. For the eighth task, four pieces of information, two of them unrelated to shopping, had to be written on a postcard (for example, the price of a pound of tomatoes) during the errands. The observers noted qualitatively any unusual performance of the tasks by the patients which reflected poor planning and organization. Although one of the patients completed all the tasks satisfactorily, errors in the execution by all three patients were related to: inefficiences, where a more effective strategy could be used; and inability to follow exactly the instructions given, for example shopping outside the allowed area and failing to pay for a newspaper. Some of the errors could be explained as motivation or memory problems. This study demonstrated the importance of the observation of patients with executive deficits resulting from traumatic brain injury in real life situations. A patient may achieve normal levels in routine task performance, but cannot organize his or her own life.

Metacognition

Metacognition is defined as: an individual's knowledge of his or her own cognitive processes and capacities, or 'knowing what you know'. The executive processes operate on this metaknowledge and allow us to monitor our own performance. Patients with frontal lobe lesions often show loss of insight or self-awareness which may be related to metacognition.

Executive functions have been linked to the retrieval of memories. Confabulation, when autobiographical memories are clearly recalled

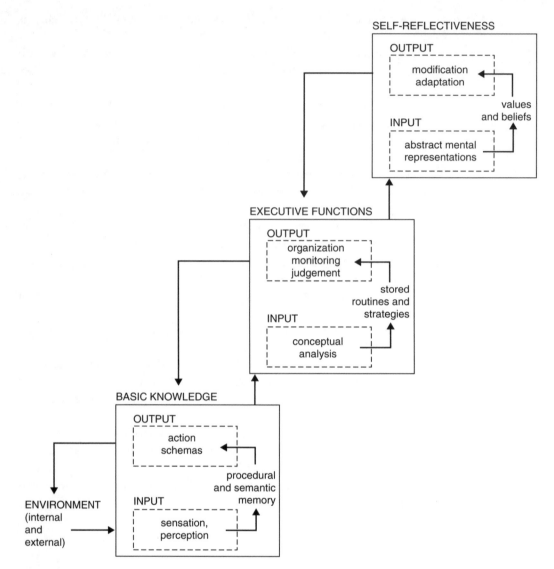

Fig. 8.3 Interaction of: basic knowledge; executive functions; and self-reflectiveness (based on Sohlberg *et al.*, 1993).

but they are untrue, is observed in some patients with frontal lobe damage and amnesia. This suggests that a verification stage linked to executive processing is part of the retrieval of memories (Shallice & Burgess, 1996).

A model of cognition developed by Sohlberg *et al.* (1993) has three levels of processing. At each level in the model, the input information is matched (comparator) with stored knowledge based on past experience. The output from each level interacts with the level below. Figure 8.3 is adapted from this model.

Sensation, basic knowledge: information from the external environment is processed in working memory and matched with stored semantic and procedural knowledge. For routine activities, the output response is then activated.

Executive functions: this level is activated when there is no matching with input conditions at the basic level. Input to the executive level of controlled processing is matched with stored plans, and routines for problem-solving. Output of this processing at the executive level feeds back down to the basic level for output response.

Self reflectiveness, metacognition: input from the executive level is matched with abstract representations of values and beliefs. Output from this feeds back down to the executive level.

The importance of metacognition in executive functioning has been recognized. However, more research is needed to develop methods of assessment and treatment of metacognitive deficits in the individual patient.

Summary

(1) The executive system directs and regulates action and behaviour. The component executive skills allow us to formulate goals, set plans and organize the responses to a new situation.

(2) Habitual behaviour is activated by environmental triggers which select appropriate stored schemas and inhibit all other schemas. This is known as contention scheduling. Flexible problem-solving in non-routine activity requires controlled executive processing by a supervisory executive system located in the frontal lobes.

(3) The executive functions operate on stored routines and strategies for organizing and correcting behaviour. The interaction with high-level metacognitive processes has been recognized.

References

Duncan, J. (1986) Disorganization of behaviour after frontal lobe damage. *Cognitive Neuropsychology* **3**(3), 271–90.

Frith, C. D., Friston, K., Liddle, P. F. & Frackowiack, R. S. J. (1991) Willed action and prefrontal cortex in man: a study with PET. *Proceedings of the Royal Society of London*, **B244**, 241–6.

Luria, A. R. (1966) *The Higher Cortical Functions in Man*. New York: Basic Books.

Norman, D. A. (1981) Categorization of action slips. *Psychological Review* **88**, 1–15.

Passingham, R. E. (1996) Attention to action. *Philosophical Transactions of the Royal Society of London* **B351**, 1473–9.

Shallice, T. (1982) Specific impairment of planning. *Philosophical Transactions of the Royal Society of London* **B298**, 199–209.

Shallice, T. & Burgess, P. W. (1991) Deficits in strategy application following frontal lobe damage in man. *Brain* **114**, 727–41.

Shallice, T. & Burgess, P. W. (1996) The domain of supervisory processes and temporal organization of behaviour. *Philosophical Transactions of the Royal Society of London* **351**, 1405–12.

Shiffrin, R. M. & Schneider, W. (1977) Controlled and automatic human information processing: II. Perceptual learning, automatic attending, and a general theory. *Psychological Review* **84**, 127–90.

Sohlberg, M. M., Mateer, C. & Stuss, D. T. (1993) Contemporary approaches to the management of executive control dysfunction. *Journal of Head Trauma Rehabilitation* **8**(1), 45–58.

Further reading

Toglia, J. P. (1991) Generalization of treatment: a multicontext approach to cognitive perceptual impairments in adults with brain injury. *American Journal of Occupational Therapy* **45**, 505–16.

Part III

Assessment of Perception and Cognition in Occupational Therapy

Chapter 9   Introduction to Assessment

Assessment in occupational therapy is an ongoing process which starts on admission in the pre-treatment phase and extends through the treatment phase to the evaluation of treatment. Historically, assessments are based on the observation of the patient performing functional tasks in a natural environment. In the 1980s the development of more standardized assessments coincided with the need for more concrete outcome measures which communicate the effectiveness of treatment to the multi-disciplinary team. These standardized tests led to the identification of the component of perception and cognition that is impaired. The benefit of more scientific assessments, however, does sacrifice their ecological validity.

Assess occupational performance or impairment?

Two approaches to the assessment of perception and cognition, which are not mutually exclusive, will be considered.

(1) *Functional (top-down) assessment* involves the observation of the performance of activites of daily living (ADL) that are relevant to the client's lifestyle. The deficits in performance indicate the appropriate adaptations and compensation needed to improve function.
(2) *Impairment-based (bottom-up) assessment* focuses on the component skills which underlie occupational performance. Standardized tests are used to identify the perceptual or cognitive component skill that is impaired. Remedial treatment can be focused on the particular impairment that is affecting function.

The initial interview with the client leads to the formulation of hypotheses about his or her occupational dysfunction. A standardized assessment of ADL provides more information about the client's level of independence, but most ADL assessments are heavily weighted towards physical rather than cognitive dysfunction.

Functional assessment identifies the problems in task performance in a natural context. However, the client with cognitive dysfunction often presents with problems that are difficult to specify, unlike the more overt problems originating in physical disability. Functional assessment can be based on objective observations by the therapist, or on self-rating of performance by the client. In some cases, the carer may be the only person who can offer the required information about the client's behaviour.

Impairment can be measured by tests which cover all areas of perception and cognition. The impairment is easier to quantify and the results can be clearly communicated to the members of the multidisciplinary team. The effect of the impairment on function can be predicted more easily when the perceptual and cognitive deficits are relatively circumscribed or discrete; for example, poor face recognition or body scheme disorder. Global deficits, on the other hand, can be seen at all levels of function; for example, memory or attention deficits can affect all activities.

The strength of the functional approach is that it reflects occupational performance in everyday life. The outcome can be supported and strengthened by identifying the impairment level across tasks. The impairment approach uses tests that are standardized and less subjective. Predictions may be made about where task performance will break down.

Figure 9.1 summarizes the assessment of function and impairment and shows how they can interact.

Choosing assessments

The choice of assessments depends on several factors including: the setting; the tools available; and the length of both the therapist's and the client's time.

The acute, hospital-based setting may involve in-patient, or short-burst out-patient, treatment. Here the assessments are often client centred, and the aim is to indicate both the potential for rehabilitation and the safety for discharge. The community setting may be long term in the client's own home, or in short out-patient visits. The focus of assessment is now on the adaptation of the client's environment, and on the changes in the client's performance over time which will indicate the rate of deterioration.

Resources are needed for the purchase of standardized test batteries and for staff training in their use. Time and money is needed for occupational therapists to become registered to use some of the

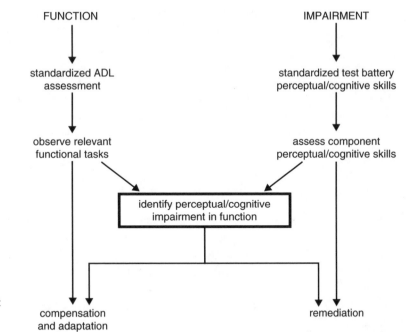

FUNCTION

standardized ADL
assessment

observe relevant
functional tasks

IMPAIRMENT

standardized test battery
perceptual/cognitive skills

assess component
perceptual/cognitive skills

identify perceptual/cognitive
impairment in function

compensation
and adaptation

remediation

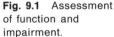

Fig. 9.1 Assessment of function and impairment.

standardized cognitive tests. A clinical psychologist in the multi-disciplinary team may provide support and advice. Simple objective tests can be made at the bedside and may provide early indications of cognitive problems. In a study of the assessment tools used by head-injured patients (Haig, 1997), 96% of the occupational therapists used both standardized and non-standardized assessments during the early rehabilitation stage.

When time is limited, a functional assessment may be the only option, and the therapist's skill in observing cognitive problems is paramount. Observation is also a crucial part of the administration of standardized tests. The patient's behaviour during the tests can be as important as the actual scores (Jesshope *et al.*, 1991). After screening for the component skill that is impaired, the effects of this deficit in functional tasks can be observed.

Clinical reasoning, which directs and guides occupational therapy practice, must determine the ultimate choice of assessments for perception and cognition.

Pre-assessment check-list

Before embarking on any programme for the assessment of perception and cognition, the limitations of the client for the completion of the tests must be addressed.

- Establish the patient's hand dominance.
- Assess motor ability. Is the patient able to manipulate objects and use a pencil?
- Check eyesight. Does the patient require glasses for reading?
- Ask for pre-test screening by the speech and language therapist for comprehension, receptive and expressive dysphasia.
- Assessment of pre-morbid IQ from:
  ○ previous education and experience
  ○ information from relatives
  ○ National Adult Reading Test (Nelson, 1982).
- Is English a second language for the patient? Some tests require knowledge of written and spoken English.
- Assessment of attention level and distractibility – visual and auditory.
- Assess the patient's attitude to testing and his or her anxiety level.
- Look at CT scan result, if available.
- Ensure a comfortable and quiet environment for testing.
- Take into account the experience of the assessor.

Standardized tests of perception and cognition

When standardized test batteries are appropriate and available, there are advantages and disadvantages in their use.

Advantages
- The tests are objective.
- There is a clear procedure for the administration of each test.
- Tests can be repeated on the same patient at different times to show progress.
- Different therapists can assess the same patient, and reliable comparisons can be made.
- The results can be used to support and extend functional assessments.

Disadvantages
- Good patient cooperation is required.
- Some patients may not be able to complete the whole battery on one occasion without fatigue.
- Tests are mainly static displays without any time dimension and performed in the absence of context.
- It is difficult to administer some of the tests to patients with receptive language problems.

There are four standardized tests that cover most areas of perception and cognition:

- The Rivermead Perceptual Assessment Battery (RPAB)
- The Chessington Occupational Therapy Neurological Assessment Battery (COTNAB)
- The Loewenstein Occupational Therapy Cognitive Assessment (LOTCA)
- The Middlesex Elderly Assessment of Mental State (MEAMS).

The Cognitive Assessment of Minnesota (CAM) also provides a useful initial assessment, but the language used needs to be converted to straight English vocabulary.

An outline of each of the four screening tests will now be considered. The individual tests are listed in the appropriate chapters in Part III.

The Rivermead Perceptual Assessment Battery (RPAB)
(Whiting *et al.*, 1985)

The RPAB was designed for the assessment of visual and spatial perception in occupational therapy. The RPAB provides a good initial test for the screening of all patients with neurological impairment. Perceptual problems which need further assessment in functional activities can be identified. Screening for perceptual problems should be done before assessing higher cognitive functions, for example memory and executive functions.

The original RPAB was standardized on normal subjects aged 16 to 69 years (Cockburn *et al.*, 1982), and validated on a group of stroke and head injury patients. A further standard for the elderly aged 65 to 92 years has been added.

The complete battery of 16 tests takes around one hour to administer. Studies in the literature have taken failure on three (Jesshope *et al.*, 1991) or four (Edmans & Lincoln, 1987) of the subtests to indicate the presence of perceptual problems. Lincoln & Edmans (1989) investigated the possibility of a shortened version of the RPAB by analysing the scores on all the tests in 169 normal subjects and 190 stroke patients. The results of the analysis produced three shortened versions. From these, the shortened version of eight tests was chosen which was most closely related to the total score and was rated the most acceptable by the therapists. The time taken to administer the shorter version is 35 minutes on average. The shortened version was also supported by a statistical analysis of the scores of a group of stroke and traumatic brain injury patients by Matthey *et al.* (1993) who identified the subtests where maximum scores were obtained by the majority of the group.

When RPAB scores were compared with ADL assessment of a group of stroke patients at discharge, a significant relationship was found (Jesshope *et al.*, 1991; Matthey *et al.*, 1993). A clinical relationship between scores on the RPAB and performance in three functional tasks has also been shown (Donnelly *et al.*, 1998). The tasks were: setting a table for two; putting on a cardigan; and making a sandwich and packing a lunch box. A check-list of the steps in each task was compiled and the therapist assessed each step.

Chessington Occupational Therapy Neurological Assessment Battery (COTNAB)
(Tyerman *et al.*, 1986)

The COTNAB is a comprehensive assessment of neurological function for use in occupational therapy. The battery of tests, covering a wider area of abilities than the RPAB, is divided into four sections:

- visual perception
- constructional ability
- sensory–motor ability
- ability to follow instructions.

The COTNAB was originally standardized on 100 traumatic brain-injured and 50 stroke patients aged 16 to 65 years, with 50 normal controls matched for age. A second version has been developed for patients over 65 years (Laver & Huchison, 1994).

A comparison of the RPAB and COTNAB was made with a group of 16 traumatic brain injury and 16 stroke patients (Sloan *et al.*, 1991). The average time taken to administer the RPAB was 49 minutes, compared with 80 minutes for the COTNAB. The extra time needed for the COTNAB was outweighed by the additional information obtained in the section testing the ability to follow instructions which is not covered by the RPAB. The patients' subjective rating of the tests showed no preference for one of the batteries compared with the other.

Laver & Huchison (1994) asked 47 normal healthy elderly people (aged 65 to 87 years) to record their test experience of the COTNAB for factors such as interest, anxiety, difficulty and relevance on a five-point scale. The results confirmed the ability of an elderly client group to use the COTNAB for assessment.

Loewenstein Occupational Therapy Cognitive Assessment (LOTCA)
(Katz *et al.*, 1989)

The LOTCA was developed in Israel to measure cognitive function in patients aged 20 to 70 years with brain injury. The battery is divided into four sections:

- orientation
- perception
- visuomotor organization
- thinking operations.

A second version is now available which is validated for the elderly, aged 70 to 91 years. In a comparative study of American and Israeli CVA patients, no significant differences were shown between the two groups (Cermak *et al.*, 1995). This study also confirmed that the LOTCA is a valid assessment of cognitive–perceptual abilities in both right and left cerebal damage.

Middlesex Elderly Assessment of Mental State (MEAMS)

The MEAMS was developed as a screening assessment of cognitive skills in elderly people. The battery covers orientation, memory, new learning, naming, comprehension, arithmetic, visuospatial skills, perception, fluency and motor perseveration. These 12 subtests are not IQ dependent and can be completed in approximately ten minutes.

The battery was validated on a group of 120 elderly clients, aged 65 to 93 years, with conditions including Alzheimer's and multi-infarct dementia.

Other standardized tests of cognition

There are other standardized tests which focus on a specific component of cognition:

- *The Rivermead Behavioural Memory Test (RBMT)* is designed to test all areas of everyday memory.
- *The Doors and People Test* is a test of long-term memory with emphasis on the selective impairment of visual and verbal memory.

- *The Behavioural Inattention Test (BIT)* assesses unilateral visual neglect using behavioural subtests as well as conventional paper and pencil tests (Hartman-Maeir & Katz, 1995).
- *The Test of Everyday Attention (TEA)* assesses sustained attention, selective attention and attentional switching.
- *The Behavioural Assessment of Dysexecutive Syndrome (BADS)* includes tests of the cognitive skills involved in problem-solving, planning and organizing behaviour that relate to everyday life.

Summary

(1) Assessment of perception and cognition in occupational therapy can be approached in two main ways: a top-down functional assessment of daily living activities to identify cognitive problems; and a bottom-up assessment of the component cognitive skill that is impaired.

(2) Functional assessment allows the identification of cognitive problems in a realistic setting. Standardized test batteries provide valid and reliable measures of the components of perception and cognition which can be used to predict functional problems.

(3) The choice of appropriate assessments for the client with cognitive problems depends on: the available time and resources; the therapeutic setting; the ability of the client to complete the tests; and the clinical reasoning of the therapist.

References

Cermak, S. A., Katz, N., McGuire, E., Greenbaum, S., Peralta, C., Maser-Flanagan, V. (1995) Performance of Americans and Israelis with cerebrovascular accident on the Loewenstein Occupational Therapy Cognitive Assessment (LOTCA). *American Journal of Occupational Therapy* **49**(6), 500–506.

Cockburn, J., Bhavnani, G., Whiting, S. & Lincoln, N. B. (1982) Normal performance on some tests of perception in adults. *British Journal of Occupational Therapy* **45**, 67–8.

Donnelly, S. M., Hextell, D. & Matthey, S. (1998) The Rivermead Perceptual Assessment Battery: its relationship to selected functional activities. *British Journal of Occupational Therapy* **61**(1), 27–32.

Edmans, J. & Lincoln, N. B. (1987) The frequency of perceptual deficits after stroke. *Clinical Rehabilitation* **1**, 273–81.

Haig, J. (1997) Assessment tools used by occupational therapists with head-injured patients in a rehabilitation setting. *British Journal of Occupational Therapy* **60**(12), 541–5.

Hartman-Maeir, A. & Katz, N. (1995) Validity of the Behavioural Inattention Test (BIT): relationships with functional tasks. *American Journal of Occupational Therapy* **49**(6), 507–516.

Jesshope, J. H., Clark, M. S. & Smith, D. S. (1991) The RPAB: its application to stroke patients and relationship with function. *Clinical Rehabilitation* **5**, 115–22.

Katz, N., Itzkowich, M., Averbuch, S. & Elazar, B. (1989) LOTCA battery for brain-injured adults: reliability and validity. *American Journal of Occupational Therapy* **43**(3), 184–92,

Laver, A. J. & Huchison, S. (1994) The performance and experience of normal elderly people on the Chessington Occupational Therapy Neurological Assessment Battery (COTNAB). *British Journal of Occupational Therapy* **57**(4), 137–42.

Lincoln, N. B. & Edmans, J. A. (1989) A shortened version of the Rivermead Perceptual Assessment Battery. *Clinical Rehabilitation* **3**, 199–204.

Matthey, S., Donelly, S. M. & Hextell, D. L. (1993) The clinical usefulness of the Rivermead Perceptual Assessment Battery: statistical considerations. *British Journal of Occupational Therapy* **56**(10), 365–70.

Nelson, H. E. (1982) *The National Adult Reading Test*. Windsor: NFER-Nelson.

Sloan, R. L., Downie, C., Hornby, J. & Pentland, B. (1991) Routine screening of brain-damaged patients: a comparison of the Rivermead Perceptual Assessment Battery and the Chessington Occupational Therapy Neurological Assesment Battery. *Clinical Rehabilitation* **5**, 265–72.

Tyerman, R., Tyerman, A., Howard, P. & Hatfield, C. (1986) *The Chessington Occupational Therapy Neurological Assessment Battery*. Nottingham Rehab. Ltd.

Whiting, S., Lincoln, N. B., Bhavnani, G. & Cockburn, J. (1985) *The Rivermead Perceptual Assessment Battery*. Windsor: NFER-Nelson.

Chapter 10   Visual Perceptual Deficits and Agnosia

The patient with visual perceptual deficits is often unaware of any problem. Function is below the expected levels, even though there may be no sensory loss or muscle weakness. When objects are only partially exposed to view, or are seen from unusual angles, there is difficulty in recognizing them (Bechinger & Tallis, 1986). The classic study in rehabilitation, which recognized a relationship between disturbance of visual perception and performance in activities of daily living in left hemiplegic patients, was made by Lorenze & Cancro (1962). The importance of visual perception for effective performance and, more crucially, for safety was later identified by Diller & Weinberg (1970).

Poor object or face recognition is most common in patients with posterior lesions. Tasks which use several objects are most affected. The ability to recognize objects from touch or from a verbal description gives further information about the recognition processing of the particular individual. Face recognition problems affect a person's independence, particularly in relation to social interaction.

Visual perceptual deficits may be underlying any cognitive deficit and they should form part of the initial screening. The assessment may be complicated by double vision in multiple sclerosis, and by poor coordination of eye movements in traumatic brain injury.

The standardized test batteries described in Chapter 9 include individual tests of visual perception, and object and face recognition. Both standardized and functional assessments will be described in this chapter under the headings of basic visual perception, visual object agnosia and face recognition problems. Spatial deficits, which are closely linked to visual perception, will be described in Chapter 11, together with a description of visual field and eye movements.

Deficits in basic visual perception

The basic visual features which form the perceptual analysis of objects are colour, shape, size, depth, object constancy and figure ground.

Tactile, auditory and olfactory input also contribute to the perceptual analysis.

A form board can be used as an initial screening test for discrimination of shape and colour (Fig. 10.1). The patient is asked to fit coloured wooden shapes of different form into corresponding shapes on the board.

Colour

Inability to recognize colour, in the absence of retinal defects, is known as achromatopsia, or colour agnosia. The patient with colour agnosia is unable to match colours, or sort different shades of the same colour. In its severe form, which occurs in bilateral posterior lesions, the visual environment is seen as black, white or grey. Some loss of colour discrimination, particularly in the blue end of the spectrum, is common in cerebral lesions (Meadows, 1974). An apparent loss of colour perception in the right hemiplegic patient is more likely to be due to a colour-naming problem.

If colour perception is impaired, faces and common objects can usually be recognized from other features, but problems arise in the use of money when bronze and silver coins appear the same. In sorting out clothes, the patient relies on tactile cues, and cannot colour-match or coordinate separate items. There is difficulty in distinguishing foods in jars, and in the selection of items, such as tins of soup or beans, from a shelf in the supermarket. Mistakes are only realized from the smell and the taste of food when the tin is opened.

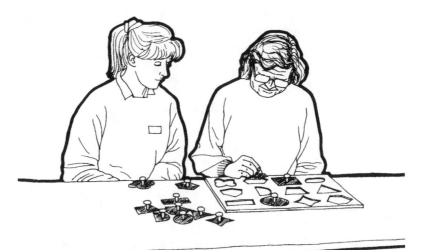

Fig. 10.1 Assessment of shape perception using a form board.

Form constancy

Form constancy is the feature of visual perception that allows us to recognize shapes and objects as the same when presented in a variety of conditions. Size is part of form constancy. The same items seen in different sizes need to be recognized as the same.

Patients with deficits in form constancy have difficulty in recognizing familiar items or objects, when they appear in unusual orientation, and without a background. There may be difficulty in selecting the appropriate item and using it correctly. In dressing, a garment may not be recognized if it is upside down or inside out, for example pants may be placed over the head.

Figure ground

Deficits in the perception of figure ground mean that objects cannot be isolated from the surfaces they are lying on, and from other objects which overlap them. The patient has difficulty in finding things. He or she cannot find the soap in the bathroom, a comb in a drawer, or a cup in a cupboard. In dressing, items of clothing cannot be isolated from the bedcover they are lying on, especially a white vest lying on a white sheet.

Sequencing

Visual perception forms the basis for semantic processing of the meaning of items in the environment. Patients with visual perceptual deficits have difficulty in following a logical sequence of images because they cannot understand the content of each part of the series. Sequencing of actions is more likely to have a basis at the level of the action production system (see Chapter 7).

Assessment

Standardized

RPAB
3 and 4 – colour matching, size recognition.
8 – figure-ground discrimination (Fig. 10.2).
9 – sequencing (Fig. 10.3).

COTNAB
Section 1, Tests I and II – overlapping figures, hidden figures.
Section 1, Test III – sequencing.

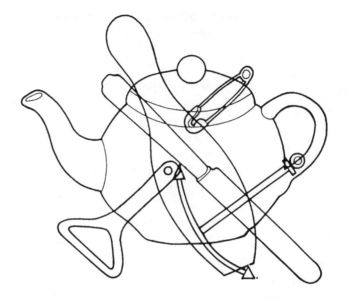

Fig. 10.2 Figure ground discrimination. RPAB 8, main picture card. Extract (not actual size) from Rivermead Perceptual Assessment Battery by permission of NFER-NELSON (all rights reserved).

LOTCA

B 4, 5 and 6 – shape identification, overlapping figures, object constancy.

Functional

Colour and shape matching

Ask the patient to:

Select items for the same colour and the same size, for example tins of food in the kitchen cupboard or on the shelves of a supermarket.

Figure ground

Observe the ability to select objects in view:

- Dressing – Find a shirt in a pile of clothes
  Point to the buttons, the sleeve, the collar
- Kitchen – Find an item in a cupboard
  Point to an electric socket on the wall
  Pick out the spoons in a drawer of cutlery.

Depth

Lay out common objects on a table in front of the patient.

Ask the patient to point to: the furthest away, the furthest to the side, and so on.

Observe the patient in activities that require estimation of depth: for example, pouring water from a jug into a glass with the unaffected hand; and walking across busy roads.

Depth perception is part of spatial perception and this is discussed further in Chapter 11.

Visual object agnosia

Agnosia is the inability to recognize familiar objects in the absence of any sensory impairment. Agnosia means literally 'no knowledge', and pure agnosia is clinically rare. Cases of pure visual object agnosia have been reported and one case study is described in detail by Humphreys & Riddoch (1987).

Visual object agnosia was first divided into two main types by Lissauer in 1900 and later supported by group studies of patients with right or left parietal lobe lesion (Warrington & Taylor, 1978; Warrington, 1982). The two types are as follows:

- *Apperceptive agnosia* is a failure to recognize objects as the result of visual perceptual impairment. Patients who are unable to copy drawings of objects, or to match objects, have object recognition problems based on impairment of visual perception in the right hemisphere.
- *Associative (semantic) agnosia* is the inability to recognize familiar objects when visual perception is intact. These agnosic patients, who are able to copy figures and name objects from verbal descriptions of their structure, cannot describe the function of objects due to impairment of semantic processing of objects in the left hemisphere.

Recent studies in cognitive neuropsychology have identified variations of these types of visual object agnosia within the two main divisions. The single case studies which relate to them are described in Parkin (1996).

The relationship between visual perceptual deficits and the performance of activities in daily living (ADL) in stroke patients has been investigated in occupational therapy (Bernspång *et al.*, 1987; Edmans & Lincoln, 1990; Titus *et al.*, 1991). The nature and the number of the perceptual tests used in each of the studies is different but, overall, the results predict that the presence of visual perceptual deficits in right or left hemisphere lesion patients will affect ADL performance adversely. Visual agnosia can be differentiated from a visual memory deficit. Patients with both these impairments cannot name objects. If it is a memory problem he or she can describe its use, but the agnosic patient cannot.

Fig. 10.3 Sequencing – RPAB 9. Extract (not actual size) from Rivermead Perceptual Assessment Battery by permission of NFER-NELSON (all rights reserved).

Visual object recognition problems, usually combined with other perceptual problems, affect function in many ways. There may be difficulty in: recognizing personal possessions, such as the contents of a handbag; choosing items in supermarket shopping; selecting the correct tools in manipulative tasks; and enjoying the abundance of flowers in a garden.

Assessment

Standardized

RPAB
2, 6 and 7 – object matching, animal halves, missing article.

COTNAB
Section 1, Test III – sequencing, includes recognition of the same object in different views and when only part of the object is seen.
Section 2, Test I – 2D construction.

LOTCA
B 3 – object identification.
C 10 – reproduction of 2D model.

Functional
- Observation of tasks involving several objects.
  Does the task break down because of inappropriate use of each object in the task?
  Is performance in the task changed by using familiar/unfamiliar objects?
- Single object recognition.
  A collection of everyday objects are hidden from the patient and are presented individually. The patient is asked to:
  o   identify each object when each is presented randomly in different views;
  o   describe the use of each object.

Tactile, auditory and olfactory agnosia

Tactile agnosia or *astereognosis* is the inability to recognize objects by touch in the presence of normal sensation, but with vision occluded.

Patients with tactile agnosia have difficulty when activities have to been done out of view. Doing up a back zip or finding coins in a pocket are examples of this. Work activities using equipment and machines often involve manipulative operations out of view.

Assessment

COTNAB

Section 3, Test I – stereognosis/tactile discrimination.

Auditory agnosia is the inability to recognize familiar sounds or to distinguish between different sounds. A patient with auditory agnosia does not distinguish the voices of different people. He or she may leave the vacuum cleaner or the TV on, and complain that his or her hearing aid is broken. Cooperation with the speech and language therapist is important.

If auditory agnosia occurs only on one side, it may be part of unilateral neglect which is described in Chapter 12.

Olfactory agnosia is the inabilty to recognize familiar smells. This has implications for safety when the smell of gas, of smoke, and of burnt food is ignored.

Face recognition problems

Prosopagnosia is the inability to recognize familiar faces. This is a deficit in visual processing of faces; even close relatives may not be recognized.

The additional processing of facial expressions and facial speech (lip-reading) makes the recognition of faces different from objects. Evidence for separate processing of faces comes from the monkey brain where cells in the temporal lobe respond selectively to faces (Perrett *et al.*, 1992).

Patients with prosopagnosia are able to identify a face as a face, and know that there is a difference between two faces, but cannot recognize who it is. Impairment at the level of the face recognition units (see Chapter 3) leads to appreciation that the face is familiar but he or she cannot be recognized. Identification of the individual person is achieved at the level of the person identity nodes. Interaction at this level with expression analysis means that relatives and close friends may be recognized from their voices and their facial expressions.

Prosopagnosia is distinguished from a memory problem by the intact knowledge of the same person in other ways, for example talking about the person by name. A patient who cannot learn the names of hospital staff may have a severe memory problem rather than poor face recognition.

Assessment

Standardized
RPAB 10 – Body (image) scheme, (b) parts of the face.

Functional
Match and/or identify photographs of family, friends and hospital staff. In the absence of language problems, pick out a named person.
Recognize family and friends in a social environment.

Summary of brain areas

The following summary gives a guide to the brain areas associated with visual perceptual deficits and visual agnosias (Fig. 10.4).

- *Occipital lobe*   – hemianopia, impairment of shape, size and depth perception.
- (bilateral)   – object agnosia, prosopagnosia.
- *Right parietal lobe* –   object constancy, apperceptive agnosia, visual object agnosia.
- *Left parietal lobe* –   associative (semantic) agnosia.
- *Temporal lobe* –   prosopagnosia.

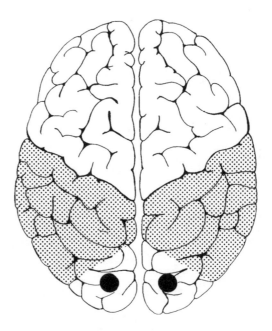

Fig. 10.4 Brain areas associated with visual perceptual deficits and agnosia.

References

Bechinger, D. & Tallis, R. (1986) Perceptual disorders in neurological disease. Part 1. *British Journal of Occupational Therapy* Sept., 282–4.

Bernspång, B., Asplund, K., Eriksson, S. & Fugi-Meyer, A. R. (1987) Motor and perceptual impairments in acute stroke patients. Effects on self-care ability. *Stroke* **18**, 1081–6.

Diller, L. & Weinberg, J. (1970) Evidence of accident-prone behaviour in hemiplegic patients. *Archives of Physical Medicine and Rehabilitation* **51**, 358–63.

Edmans, J. A. & Lincoln, N. B. (1990) The relation between perceptual deficits after stroke and independence in activities of daily living. *British Journal of Occupational Therapy* **53**, 139–42.

Humphreys, G. W. & Riddoch, M. J. (1987) *To See or Not to See: A Case Study of Visual Agnosia.* London: Lawrence Erlbaum.

Lorenze, E. & Cancro, R. (1962) Dysfunction of visual perception with hemiplegia. *Archives of Physical Medicine and Rehabilitation* **43**, 514–17.

Meadows, J. C. (1974) Disturbed perception of colours associated with localized cerebral lesion. *Brain* **97**, 615–32.

Parkin, A. J. (1996) *Explorations in Cognitive Neuropsychology.* Oxford: Blackwell.

Perrett, D. I., Hietanen, M. W., Oram, M. W. & Benson, P. J. (1992) Organization and functions of cells responsive to faces in the temporal cortex. *Philosophical Transactions of the Royal Society of London* **B335**, 23–30.

Titus, M. N. D., Gall, N. G., Yerxa, E. J., Roberson, T. A. & Mack, W. (1991) Correlation of perceptual performance and activities of daily living in stroke patients. *American Journal of Occupational Therapy* **45**, 410–18.

Warrington, E. K. (1982) Neuropsychological studies of object recognition. *Philosophical Transactions of the Royal Society of London* **B298**, 15–33.

Warrington, E. K. & Taylor, A. M. (1978) Two categorical stages in object recognition. *Perception* **7**, 695–705.

Chapter 11   Spatial Deficits

Spatial deficits can originate in basic visual perception, but the additional spatial component becomes obvious in tasks that require assembling parts together to construct a whole. Performance is also poor when the position of the parts of the body cannot be related to objects in reaching space. Problems in route-finding arise when the whole body cannot orient to the layout of far space.

In the assessment of both visual and spatial perception, any background visual field deficit, or poor scanning of space must be identified first. A global, but rare, loss of spatial relations processing in both near and far space is known as spatial relations syndrome. Unilateral neglect is spatial disorder with an overlay of attentional deficits and this will be considered in Chapter 12. In this chapter, the deficits of spatial perception will be divided into: visual field and scanning; body scheme; constructional praxis; and topographical orientation.

Visual field and scanning defects

Visual field defects

A visual field defect is a partial loss of vision which affects the perception of the space around by limiting the field of view. Visual field defects can originate at any point in the visual pathway from the optic tract at the base of the brain to the occipital lobes (see Fig. 4.2).

Hemianopia is defined as the loss of half of the visual field in one or both eyes. The term is often erroneously used since there is rarely total loss of half the visual fields. In CVA and traumatic brain injury, there is a loss of variable areas of each visual field, depending on the level and the extent of the disruption of the visual pathway. In multiple sclerosis, there may be loss of the central area of the visual field associated with demyelination of the optic nerve. Also diplopia (double vision) reduces the ability to discriminate form and affects spatial perception.

Some patients develop strategies to overcome visual field defects, by turning the head. Reading often remains a problem. In scanning the page from left to right, the patient with loss of the right visual field cannot make sense of the text after the first few words. The patient with left visual field defect cannot start to read, or has difficulty in picking up the next line as the eyes return to the left.

Scanning defects

A scanning defect is the inability to explore the space around by movements of the eyes, which includes fixation on targets and following moving targets.

Eye movements are impaired by injury to the system controlling the muscles at the back of the eye. The brain stem, together with projections from the frontal and occipital lobes, forms the oculomotor control system. Loss of control leads to poor visual scanning, and slower speed of eye movements in overt shifts of attention. Loss of the coordination of the movements of both eyes to focus on a target may lead to double vision and poor depth perception.

In patients with traumatic brain injury, the eye movements may be spontaneous and erratic. Random scanning movements lead to delay in interpreting an image. This is less common in CVA. Loss of pursuit eye movements in any or all planes means that the eyes cannot track a moving image. Computer games and many sports activities then become impossible. Poor saccadic eye movements make reading difficult. Poor scanning of one side of space should be investigated before the assessment of unilateral neglect.

Assessment

If possible, the patient should be referred for detailed examination of the visual fields using an optometer.

Spot the ball

Use a small coloured ball at the end of a black wand. The eyes are observed when the patient is asked to:

- Follow the ball as it is moved slowly in different directions – up and down, from left to right, and from right to left.
- Fixate on the ball held in one position.

Functional

The movements of the patient's eyes are observed in functional tasks, for example:

- Look at a large picture in a newspaper.
- Look for specific items in a kitchen cupboard at a named location, for example: top or bottom shelf, right or left side.

Disorders of body scheme

In body scheme disorders there is a loss of knowledge of the position of body parts and the spatial relations between them. Body image dysfunction, on the other hand, has psychosocial as well as physical components.

Body knowledge processing has several levels of representation, which results in different types of body scheme disorder. These disorders will now be discussed.

Somatognosia is a failure to recognize the parts of the body and to perceive their relative positions in space. The patient with somatognosia has poor balance and equilibrium. Movements are inaccurate, even though proprioception is normal.

Right/left discrimination deficit is the inability to distinguish right and left in the symmetrical parts of the body. Confusion of right and left may be part of somatognosia. Many normal subjects have difficulty in right/left discrimination, particularly when asked to point to parts of body shapes presented in unconventional orientations.

Anosognosia is the denial of the severity or even the presence of an affected limb. When asked to move the limb, the commands are often ignored, and various reasons are offered as an excuse. One patient called his arm George after his son who didn't work! Also the patient is in danger of injury to the limb. Anosognosia may be part of severe unilateral neglect (see Chapter 12), or part of a body scheme disorder together with proprioceptive sensory loss and other cognitive impairments.

Autopagnosia is an inability to identify the parts of the body. Finger agnosia is when this is only related to the fingers. Both of these may be a naming problem associated with aphasia.

Body scheme disorder is not a single deficit and may present in different forms. Some authors have described syndromes which include one aspect of body scheme. The loss of body scheme may be bilateral, or it may affect one side of the body in the form of unilateral neglect.

Assessments have been developed to identify different aspects of body scheme disorder. Corbett & Shah (1996) describe seven tests and they conclude that further studies are needed to validate them.

The test of body scheme that is most commonly used in occupational therapy asks the patient to draw, or to assemble a model of, the parts of the body in the correct relationship to each other. If drawing is difficult, pointing to the body parts on a model, or on the patient's own body, can be used. Pointing to body parts by imitation of the therapist has difficulties in transferring the instructions from the therapist's body to that of the patient, if they are facing.

Body scheme disorder is common in stroke patients (McDonald, 1960) but there have been few studies of the relationship between this deficit and ADL assessments. Studies of groups of stroke patients by McDonald (1960) and Warren (1981) showed a correlation between body scheme deficits and performance in: bathing and self-care; and upper extremity dressing; respectively. The impact of loss of body scheme on reading and writing is significant for some patients (Van Deusen, 1993).

The small number of studies in neuropsychology have indicated that body scheme disorder is linked to damage of the parietal and temporal lobes.

The only standardized test of body scheme is in the Rivermead Perceptual Assessment Battery (RPAB) (Fig. 11.1). In an analysis of the subtests of the RPAB for clinical usefulness (Matthey *et al.*, 1993), the body image and self-identification tests were among the five subtests that were most sensitive to detect change.

Assessment _____

Standardized
RPAB 10a – Body scheme (Fig. 11.1).
RPAB 16 – Self-identification.

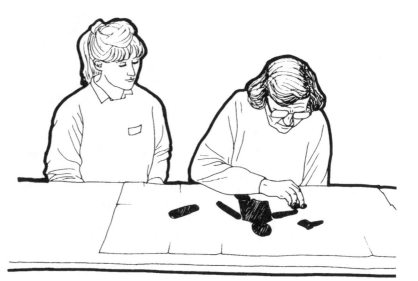

Fig. 11.1 Assessment of body scheme – RPAB 10a. Extract (not actual size) from Rivermead Perceptual Assessment Battery by permission of NFER–NELSON (all rights reserved).

General body scheme can be assessed as follows:
The therapist sits to the side of the patient and asks him or her to:

- point to body parts on command, and by imitation;
- move a body part after the therapist has touched it;
- touch one part of the body with another part, e.g. 'touch your left ear with your right hand'.

Constructional deficits

Constructional impairment can be defined as: difficulty in the assembly of single parts into a two- or three-dimensional whole. The spatial part of the task is missed.

Constructional deficits have been reported in patients with right and left parietal, posterior and frontal lobe lesions (see Neistadt, 1990 for a list of sources). This means that nearly all adults with brain injury may have impairment of constructional ability. However, very few studies have been made of the effect of constructional deficits on performance of ADL. In a group of stroke patients, a comparative study of ADL performance using the Klein–Bell Scale (Klein & Bell, 1982) with seven perceptual tests found the most significant correlation with tests of 3D constructional praxis and block design (Titus *et al.*, 1991). A different approach was used by Donnelly *et al.* (1998), who isolated the constructional components of three functional tasks based on a task analysis. The three tasks were: making a sandwich and packing a lunch box; putting on a cardigan; and setting a table. Thirty-five stroke patients completed the RPAB and also a functional assessment using a check-list developed from constructional steps of each task. The results of the study suggested that patients with perceptual problems as assessed by the RPAB do have problems with constructional tasks.

Most of the standardized assessment batteries include tests of constructional ability. Simple copying of geometric forms is based on a developmental approach to the tests. Children from three to eight years can draw circles, squares, triangles and diamonds in ascending order of development. There is no reason to assume, however, that the recovery of perceptual function after brain damage follows the same sequence (Abreu & Toglia, 1987).

Functional assessment can be based on the observation of tasks with a large constructional component. Many domestic and DIY activities demand constructional ability, for example in the assembly of a vacuum cleaner, food mixer or electric drill. The instructions for assembly need to be visual for the right hemiplegic patient, and verbal for the left hemiplegic patient. Laying the table, putting tops on jars, and decorating a cake all have a spatial component. Constructional ability is part of many work and leisure activities, such as dressmaking and woodwork.

Constructional apraxia

Constructional apraxia is defined as difficulty in the organization of complex actions in space, either on command or spontaneously. Some authors, however, define constructional apraxia as: difficulty in producing designs in two and three dimensions, by copying, drawing, or construction (Zoltan, 1996).

This conflict in the definition of constructional apraxia may be due to the fact that it is only revealed in simple tests with paper and pencil. When single items are put together to form a whole, not only must the spatial relations of the parts be perceived accurately but also the movements must be planned and performed with spatial accuracy to achieve the whole. The link between perceptual and motor components led this deficit to be grouped with the apraxias. In Chapter 14 dyspraxia is considered in relation to task performance using objects. Constructional apraxia is now considered as a deficit revealed in tests of constructional ability which may or may not be a true apraxia. When a patient with constructional problems has difficulty in initiating the action, and perseveration occurs during the progress of the movements, the deficit may be called a type of apraxia.

Concha (1987) stated that severe constructional apraxia affects all daily living activities. A clear link has been shown between constructional apraxia and inability to dress the upper body (Baum & Hall, 1981; Warren, 1981). In the study by Warren, a two-dimensional copying task was used as the constructional test with 101 stroke patients. Baum & Hall used two- and three-dimensional copying tasks in a group of 37 patients with traumatic brain injury who had multiple lesions. In both these studies, no difference was found between right and left hemisphere lesion patients in the group. The most likely feature that distinguishes constructional apraxia from visuoperceptual disorders and from other forms of apraxia (see Chapter 14) is a loss of the integration of visuospatial and motor planning processes.

The term 'dressing apraxia' has been used to describe the inability to dress oneself. Task analysis of dressing reveals that many perceptual and cognitive components are involved:

Stage	Perceptual/cognitive component
Select garment	Colour, figure ground, form constancy
Orient garment in space	Spatial perception, right/left discrimination
Orient garment to body	Body scheme
Put garment on	Body scheme, constructional praxis
All stages	Attention to right and left personal space, sequencing, planning, flexible problem-solving

Assessment of each of the components may identify the stage where intervention will have the greatest effect and may suggest suitable compensation strategies. Labelling top/bottom, right/left with colours or words will facilitate spatial perception. Body scheme disorder may respond to verbal strategies associated with the limb movements for the left hemiplegic patient (right hemisphere lesion).

Assessment

Standardized

RPAB 11   2D right and left copying of shapes.
RPAB 12   2D right and left copying of words.
RPAB 13   3D copying a model from component blocks (Fig. 11.2).
RPAB 14   Cube copying.

COTNAB, Section 2 (constructional ability)
I   2D construction – copy drawings.
II   3D construction – assemble a 3D model with replica blocks.
III Block printing – copying designs using printing blocks.

COTNAB, Section 4 (ability to follow instructions)
I   Construction of a wire coathanger using a standard jig. The instructions for assembly are written.
II   The assembly of a three-dimensional construction. The instructions are a series of photographs of the stages.

LOTCA, Section C (visuomotor organization)
9   Copy geometric forms.
10   Reproduction of 2D model.
11   Pegboard reconstruction.
12   Coloured block design.
13   Plain block design.
14   Reproduction of a puzzle.
15   Drawing a clock.

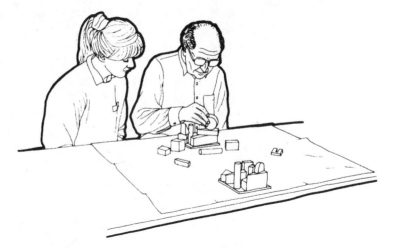

Fig. 11.2 Assessment of constructional ability – RPAB 13, 3D copying. Extract (not actual size) from Rivermead Perceptual Assessment Battery by permission of NFER–NELSON (all rights reserved).

Functional

Observe familiar tasks that have a major constructional component at an appropriate level; for example, dressing, preparing a sandwich, laying the table for two people, writing a cheque, putting up an ironing board, assembling a food mixer.

Topographical disorientation

Topographical disorientation is difficulty in finding the way in the large-scale spatial environment. This may be due to the loss of the ability to recognize the relevant landmarks. Finding the way also requires the integration of the spatial relations between body and the environment, and between landmarks irrespective of the position of the body. Assessment therefore includes landmark recognition, and the ability to move between them from start to finish.

Tests which ask patients to locate places on a map, or follow paths through a paper and pencil maze use static information in one field of view. There have been reports of patients who have topographical disorientation but who have shown no deficits in these static tests. A pilot who could not find his way in new surroundings was able to localize the main cities on a blank map of France. He could also fly an aeroplane where he had an aerial view, and the use of navigational equipment as an external aid (Habib & Sirigu, 1987). Functional assessments ask the patient to find the way in a natural environment, which may be a home, a hospital ward, a route to a friend's house or the library and so on. Depth perception, proximity judgement and right/left discrimination can be assessed on the route. Landmark recognition can be tested from photographs. Some patients do not acknowledge that they have a route-finding problem and it is important to assess the task firstly without any external aids.

Social interaction is restricted for patients who cannot find their way to the shops or to join in leisure activities. Similar problems occur in severe memory loss, therefore screening should include memory assessment. A left hemiplegic patient (right side lesion) who gets lost because he or she cannot recognize and remember familiar landmarks, may be assisted by a verbal or written description of the route. The right hemiplegic patient may draw a simple map. If the problem is spatial (allocentric) in origin, and right/left discrimination is poor, the emphasis on the recognition of landmarks may prove a more successful strategy in rehabilitation.

Some patients with topographical disorientation have other perceptual problems, which may include basic impairment of depth perception, defective scanning and attention to space, or poor face recognition. However, selective impairment of topographical orientation has been reported. A case study by Habib & Sirigu (1987) described a patient with a focal lesion of the right temporal lobe, related to the inferior branches of the posterior cerebral artery, which resulted in a left hemianopia and topographical disorientation, but no other neuropsychological deficits. The involvement of the temporal lobe, and the hippocampus in particular, has been confirmed by neuro-imaging studies in patients after unilateral (either right or left) temporal lobe surgery for intractable epilepsy (Maguire *et al.*, 1996).

Assessment

Functional

Following a route
Select a simple route in a ward, the home, a familiar supermarket (Fig. 11.3) or in a workplace. The patient walks round the route and the therapist observes the errors made.

Screening check-list: depth perception, proximity judgement, right/left discrimination and recognition of landmarks.

Spatial relations syndrome

Spatial relations syndrome is a severe spatial deficit which includes the loss of perception of figure ground, form constancy, depth and distance in both near and far space.

The patient may trip up the kerb of pavements, and drop utensils off the edge of working surfaces or tables. There may be difficulty in distinguishing the top, bottom, inside and outside of clothing.

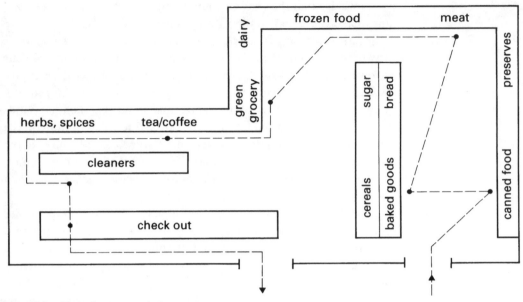

Fig. 11.3   Plan of supermarket.

A wheelchair patient may have problems in transferring when he or she cannot judge the distance between the wheelchair and the toilet or the bed. Wheelchair training is very difficult as the patient cannot estimate distances, or turn to the right or the left appropriately. The ambulant patient cannot find the way from one location to another.

A small number of severe cases of spatial relations syndrome have been reported in the literature in patients with bilateral parieto-occipital lesions (DeRenzi, 1982). Assessment of spatial relations syndrome involves testing all the components of spatial abilities described in this chapter.

Summary of brain areas

The following summary gives a guide to the brain areas associated with spatial deficits (Fig. 11.4).

- *Parietal lobe* (right) – constructional deficits (spatial).
  - body scheme disorder (anosognosia).
  - topographical disorientation.
  - spatial relations syndrome.
  (left) – constructional apraxia.
  - body scheme disorder (somatognosia).

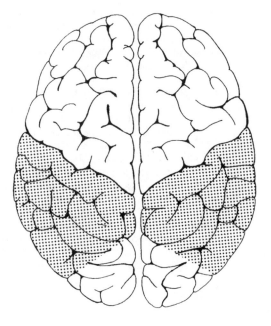

Fig. 11.4 Brain areas associated with deficits in constructional ability, body scheme and topographical orientation (temporal lobe not shown).

- *Occipito-parietal* – spatial relations syndrome.
  (bilateral)
- *Temporal lobe* – topographical disorientation.

References

Abreu, B. C. & Toglia, J. P. (1987) Cognitive rehabilitation. A model for occupational therapy. *American Journal of Occupational Therapy* **41**, 439–48.

Baum, B. & Hall, K. M. (1981) Relationship between constructional apraxia and dressing in the head-injured adult. *American Journal of Occupational Therapy* **35**, 438–42.

Concha, M. E. (1987) A review of apraxia. *British Journal of Occupational Therapy* **50**(7), 222–6.

Corbett, A. & Shah, S. (1996) Body scheme disorders following stroke and assessment in occupational therapy. *British Journal of Occupational Therapy* **59**(7), 325–9.

DeRenzi, E. (1982) *Disorders of Space Exploration and Cognition*. New York: Wiley.

Donnelly, S. M., Hextell, D. L. & Matthey, S. (1998) The Rivermead Perceptual Assessment Battery: its relationship to selected functional activities. *British Journal of Occupational Therapy* **61**, 27–32.

Habib, M. & Sirigu, A. (1987) Pure topographical disorientation: a definition and anatomical basis. *Cortex* **23**, 73–85.

Klein, R. M. & Bell, B. (1982) Self-care skills: behavioural measurement with Klein–Bell ADL scale. *Archives of Physical Medicine and Rehabilitation* **62**, 335–8.

Maguire, E. A., Burke, T., Phillips, J. & Staunton, H. (1996) Topographical disorientation following unilateral temporal lobe lesions in humans. *Neuropsychologia* **34**, 993–1001.

Matthey, S., Donnelly, S. M. & Hextell, D. L. (1993) The clinical usefulness of the Rivermead Perceptual Assessment Battery. *British Journal of Occupational Therapy* **56**, 365–70.

McDonald, J. C. (1960) An investigation of body scheme in adults with cerebral vascular accidents. *American Journal of Occupational Therapy* **14**, 75–9.

Neistadt, E. (1990) A critical analysis of occupational therapy approaches for perceptual deficits in adults with brain injury. *American Journal of Occupational Therapy* **44**, 299–304.

Titus, M. N. D., Gall, N. G., Yerxa, E. J., Roberson, T. A. & Mack, W. (1991) Correlation of perceptual performance and activities of daily living in stroke patients. *American Journal of Occupational Therapy* **45**, 410–18.

Van Deusen, J. (1993) *Body Image and Perceptual Dysfunction in Adults.* Philadelphia: Saunders.

Warren, M. (1981) Relationship of body scheme disorders to dressing performance in adult CVA. *American Journal of Occupational Therapy* **35**, 431–7.

Zoltan, B. (1996) *Vision, Perception and Cognition.* New Jersey: Slack Inc.

Chapter 12   Disorders of Attention

Disorders of attention often present a major problem in the rehabilitation of the patient with cerebral damage. A low level of arousal and alertness is common in traumatic brain injury (TBI), especially in the early stages after onset. Poor selective attention results in distractibility which affects all cognitive function. Tasks which are normally performed automatically become effortful and the patient has difficulty in responding to novel situations.

Attention controls the processing of the input of visuospatial and verbal information in working memory, and it is also involved in coding and retrieval in long-term memory. This close link between memory and attention means that some apparent memory problems may be due to an underlying attentional problem.

Poor functional performance may originate from hemi-inattention (unilateral neglect), particularly in the left hemiplegic patient (right-side lesion). Stimuli in the visual or other modalities on the one side of space (usually the left) are ignored. This deficit often resolves in a short period of time, but the persistence of severe unilateral neglect is a major factor in the failure of the left hemiplegic patient to respond to rehabilitation (Denes *et al.*, 1982).

Disorders of attention will be considered in two sections: the effects on everyday function; and the particular features of the neglect syndrome.

Deficits in everyday attention

Deficits in sustained, selective and divided attention have different effects on everyday function. These will now be discussed in turn.

Sustained attention

Arousal and alertness are the underlying attention mechanisms for sustained attention. Motivation and emotional state each have an effect on alertness. Poor sustained attention processing is most severe in patients with right prefrontal lesions.

Reduced arousal is common following the resolution of coma after TBI. External stimulation from the environment needs to be controlled to maintain arousal at an appropriate level. When the alerting mechanisms are impaired, the initiation of movement is a problem. Also, only simple tasks, which have a clearly defined goal reached in a short time, can be performed.

Poor attention span is seen in many patients with cerebral damage. Tasks that are normally performed automatically over a period of time require controlled effort and frequent cueing to maintain an adequate level of attention.

Selective attention

Selective attention is the process whereby a person attends to certain environmental stimuli in preference to others. Patients with selective attention deficit cannot filter out background noise and irrelevant visual stimuli. This attention deficit is associated with lesions of the orienting system in the right parietal lobe.

Selective attention can be subdivided into two types in relation to the attention demands of the particular activity (Wood, 1992). Some tasks require a conscious focus of attention, for example reading a newspaper in a room with other people talking. Distractibility is a common feature of selective attention deficit in this type of task and environmental control becomes a priority. Routine tasks, on the other hand, involve selective attention that is automatic, for example brushing the hair. Patients with a deficit in this type of selective attention can perform routine tasks in a familiar environment but cannot respond to changes in the task or in the setting. They are unable to suppress automatic behaviour.

Divided attention

Divided attention is the ability to perform more than one task at the same time. This places large demands on the overall attention capacity of the brain which is often reduced after cerebral damage. Two tasks that use the same sensory modality are most difficult. Listening to someone talking while following a radio programme should be avoided.

After traumatic brain injury and stroke, former routine tasks become effortful and require higher-level focused attention. Also alertness and arousal may be at a low level. The environment needs to be controlled for the optimum performance of one task at a time.

Assessment ————————————————————————

Standardized

Test of Everyday Attention (TEA)
There are eight subtests based on everyday materials.
Individual tests are designed to test one of the components of
everyday attention.

Sustained attention – test 2, elevator counting; and test 8,
            lottery.
Selective attention   – test 1, map search; and test 3, elevator
            counting with distraction.
Attention switching – tests 4, 5 and 6, visual elevator, auditory
            elevator with reversal, telephone search.
Divided attention   – test 7, telephone search dual task.

LOTCA
There is no specific subtest for attention, but an observation-
based score of attention and concentration is included. This
approach can be adopted when other standardized tests of perception and cognition are used.

Functional

Observation check-list
Sensory systems affected: visual, auditory, tactile.
Components of attention: sustained, selective, divided.
Time of day: morning, afternoon, evening.
Setting: familiar, unfamiliar.
Routine/non-routine tasks.
Memory problems: visual, verbal, delayed recall.
Select relevant functional tasks and establish baseline per-
formance.

The neglect syndrome

Neglect is defined as failure to report, respond or orient to stimuli in
the space contralateral to the site of brain lesion. Unilateral neglect is
most frequently seen in right parietal lesion which leads to left-side
neglect. There is conflicting evidence in the literature on the incidence
of right-side neglect. This may be accounted for by early resolution of
the problem or the inability to report it in left parietal lesion patients.

Unilateral neglect must not be confused with a primary visual
sensory deficit or left visual field defect. Screening for a visual field

defect is important (see Chapter 11). Some patients with unilateral visual neglect do have a visual field defect which is compensated by moving the head, but others do not.

When primary visual sensation is normal, neglect patients often show extinction to two visual stimuli, applied one on either side, simultaneously. When both hands or both sides of the face are touched, with the eyes closed, the patient with neglect may only report the stimulus on one side. In visual extinction, if one object is placed in the left visual field, or in the right visual field, it is reported. If two different objects are placed simultaneously, one in each visual field, only the object in the right field is reported.

When a patient with neglect is asked to complete a simple form board test, only the shapes on the right side of the board will be completed. If the shapes are distributed on either side at the start, only those on the right will be attempted (Fig. 12.1).

Neglect can occur in different modalities. In auditory neglect, the patient does not respond to sounds on the neglected side, even though hearing is normal.

The patient who does not explore one side of space may have:

● poor visual scanning
● hemi-inattention to visual, auditory or tactile stimuli
● loss of body scheme (see Chapter 4)
● inability to initiate movements to the contralesional side (directional hypokinesia) (see Chapter 5).

Unilateral neglect can affect all self-care, domestic and leisure activities. Poor progress towards independence in self-care alone is a major hurdle in rehabilitation. Less severe forms of neglect affect cooking, entertaining, gardening and social activities. An ambulant or wheelchair patient may always follow a route turning to the right, or bump into things on the left. The prospects for return to work are poor.

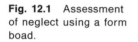

Fig. 12.1 Assessment of neglect using a form boad.

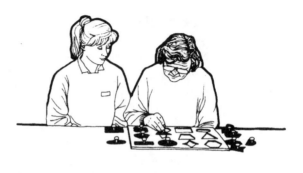

A questionnaire study of the everyday problems of patients with unilateral neglect showed that patients did not report more problems than non-neglect patients (Towle & Lincoln, 1991). However, the response from relatives showed that the neglect patients were having significantly more problems.

Conventional assessments for unilateral neglect include two-dimensional pencil and paper tests. When the patient is asked to bisect a line, there is a tendency to estimate the midpoint away from the affected side. In cancellation tasks, when the patient is asked to cross out the target numbers, letters or words, only those on the unaffected side are marked. In copying or drawing figures, one side of the outline is omitted, as in Fig. 12.2. The conventional tests are useful in the diagnosis of unilateral neglect.

Van Deusen (1988) identified the need for research studies that correlate scores in conventional tests with the performance of functional activities of all types in patients with unilateral neglect. For example, does the omission of the left side observed in shopping, gardening and self-care activities relate to scores on a line bisection test?

The Behavioural Inattention Test (BIT) is divided into conventional and behavioural tests. This standardized battery of tests was developed by Wilson *et al.* (1987) and validated on a group of 80 stroke patients and 50 controls. The behavioural tests in this battery use stimuli that are related to real life situations, for example telephone dialling and coin sorting, and they can highlight the presence of neglect that is task specific.

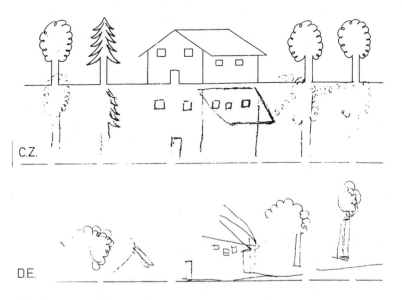

Fig. 12.2 Copying of a drawing (shown at the top) by two patients with right brain damage. Reproduced from Gainotti *et al.* (1986) *Brain* **109**, 599–612 by permission of Oxford University Press.

The original version of the BIT does not include typical self-care items but a shortened version, modified for use with acute stroke patients, was validated against assessment of neglect in self-care tasks in occupational therapy (Stone *et al.*, 1991). In a different study of right CVA patients with or without unilateral neglect (Hartman-Maeir & Katz, 1995), the behavioural subtests of picture scanning (a plate of food) and map navigation did not correlate with eating and mobility respectively, suggesting that they are not valid measures of these activities. The subtests of article reading and telling the time did not discriminate between those with and without unilateral neglect in the group. An additional factor of years of education may have influenced these scores. The other behavioural tests in the battery did show good correlation between test scores and function.

Before the assessment of unilateral neglect, the presence or absence of visual scanning and visual field defects should be identified.

Assessment

Standardized

Behavioural Inattention Test (BIT)
This battery contains six conventional pencil and paper subtests, and nine behavioural subtests.
Conventional tests include: line bisection, cancellation tasks and right/left copying. Figure 12.3 shows the star cancellation task. Behavioural tests: picture scanning, telephone dialling, menu reading, newspaper article reading, telling and setting the time, coin sorting, address and sentence copying, map navigation and card sorting.

RPAB
11 and 12 – Right/left copying shapes and words.
15   – Cancellation task.

COTNAB
2 I   – 2D construction: line bisection, copy four shapes, draw a clock, a man, a house.

Functional

Observation check-list
Observe the neglect of the left side of space in:
Self-maintenance tasks: washing, dressing and feeding.
Mobility: bumps into things on left, only turns to the right.
Reading and writing: one half of the page.
Social: only interacts with persons on the right side.

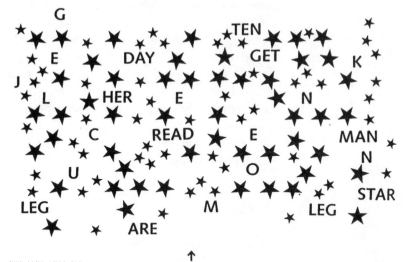

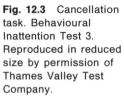

Fig. 12.3 Cancellation task. Behavioural Inattention Test 3. Reproduced in reduced size by permission of Thames Valley Test Company.

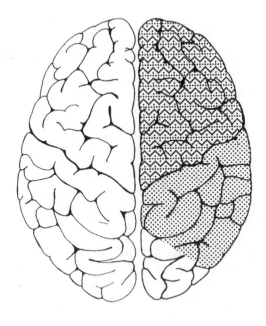

Fig. 12.4 Brain areas associated with deficits in everyday attention and unilateral neglect (temporal lobe not shown).

Summary of brain areas

The brain areas associated with sustained, selective and divided attention, and unilateral neglect are shown in Fig. 12.4.

- *Right parietal lobe* (mainly right) — selective attention deficit, unilateral neglect.
- *Temporal lobes* — auditory selective attention deficit, auditory unilateral neglect.
- *Frontal lobe* (right) — pre-motor neglect.
  — sustained attention deficit.
- *Fronto-thalamic and brain stem* — sustained attention deficit.

References

Denes, G., Semenza, C., Stoppa, E. & Lis, A. (1982) Unilateral spatial neglect and recovery from hemiplegia. A follow-up study. *Brain* **105**, 543–52.

Gainotti, G., D'Erme, P., Monteleone, D. & Silveri, M. C. (1986) Mechanisms of unilateral spatial neglect in relation to laterality of cerebral lesions. *Brain* **109**, 599–612.

Hartman-Maeir, A. & Katz, N. (1995) Validity of the Behavioural Inattention Test (BIT): relationships with functional tasks. *American Journal of Occupational Therapy* **49**, 507–16.

Stone, S. P., Wilson, B., Wroot, A., Halligan, P. W., Lange, L. S., Marshall, J. C. & Greenwood, R. J. (1991) The assessment of visuospatial neglect after acute stroke. *Journal of Neurology, Neurosurgery & Psychiatry* **54**, 345–50.

Towle, D. & Lincoln, N. (1991) Development of a questionnaire for detecting everyday problems in stroke patients with unilateral neglect. *Clinical Rehabilitation* **5**, 135–40.

van Deusen, J. (1988) Unilateral neglect: suggestions for research by occupational therapists. *American Journal of Occupational Therapy* **42**, 441–8.

Wilson, B., Cockburn, J. & Halligan, P. (1987) Development of a behavioural test of visuospatial neglect. *Archives of Physical Medicine* **68**, 98–102.

Wood, R. L. (1992) Disorders of attention: their effect on behaviour, cognition and rehabilitation. In *Clinical Management of Memory Problems* (B. A. Wilson & N. Moffat, eds), pp. 216–42. London: Chapman & Hall.

Further reading

Robertson, I. H. & Marshall, J. C. (1993) *Unilateral Neglect: Clinical and Experimental Studies*. Hove: Lawrence Erlbaum.

Chapter 13 Memory Problems

Many people with neurological deficits have some form of memory impairment. The effects of memory loss on function are varied and individual, depending on the person's lifestyle and the presence or absence of other cognitive impairment.

For some patients, the awareness of memory failures in daily living is frustrating for themselves and their family or carers. If memories of the past cannot be recalled, there is a loss of self-identity and of the pleasure of sharing past experiences.

A return to work for the memory-impaired person depends on matching the cognitive demands of the work with the spared memory of the individual. New learning is difficult and this becomes a hurdle in moving to a new job or to a different home environment where new ways of doing tasks must be learnt. Spared procedural memory retains the possibility of leisure pursuits, although support may be needed for some aspects, such as scoring.

Apparent memory loss may be related to underlying perceptual or attentional deficits. The adaptation of the environment to reduce distraction, or the development of strategies to increase alertness, may make a significant change to memory function.

Occupational therapists have the opportunity to observe and assess memory problems that relate to functional ability (Robinson, 1992). The assessment of memory can form the basis for the choice of memory aids and appropriate adaptation of the environment to optimize the patient's remaining memory function.

Working memory deficits

Working memory is the stage of memory processing, which lasts a few seconds, between the input of sensory information from the environment and the registration processing in long-term memory. It should be noted that working memory is not the same as the term 'short-term memory' which is often used clinically to mean recent memory of the previous few minutes or hours.

Working memory deficit can affect communication, finding our way around and shopping. In speaking and reading, a few words at a time are rehearsed subvocally in the phonological loop, before output in speech or passing on to long-term verbal memory. In following a route, visual images of landmarks are held for a brief time in the visuospatial sketchpad and compared with long-term visual memory for recognition. The mental arithmetic which is part of checking the change in shopping involves working memory to manipulate and rehearse small groups of numbers. Telephone numbers now require the rehearsal of around 11 numbers in working memory before dialling.

Working memory is very often normal in patients with impaired long-term memory. This selective impairment is the main evidence to support the separation of short-term and long-term memory systems. Patients with Korsakoff-type amnesia have a severely impaired long-term memory, but they can hold a conversation and they can recall numbers if there is no delay after seeing them. Deficits in working memory can be modality specific. Patients may not be able to recall numbers or words that are heard, but can recall the same information when it is presented visually.

Neuro-imaging studies have shown that the active brain areas in working memory function are anatomically widely distributed. In a PET scan study of normal subjects performing verbal tasks, the phonological store was localized in the supra marginal gyrus of the left parietal lobe, and the articulatory loop for rehearsal in Broca's area of the frontal lobe (Paulesu et al., 1993) (see Figure 1.2). In another study involving spatial memory, increased cerebral blood flow was recorded in the right parietal and right prefrontal cortex (Jonides et al., 1993).

Assessment

Digit span

A short sequence of numbers is read at the rate of one digit per second. The numbers must be repeated back in the same order. The number of digits in the sequence is increased until errors occur or a maximum of eight is reached.

Backwards digit span: the same procedure is followed but the numbers are reported in reverse order.

Normal span is seven, plus or minus two digits.

Functional

In observation of functional activities, identify problems with: handling money, using the telephone, reading a newspaper, holding a conversation, finding the way around the ward or his or her own home.

Discussion with the family and/or carer for more information.

Visual and verbal memory

An important feature of memory assessment in occupational therapy is to separate the relative loss of visual and verbal memory. The overall processing of visual and verbal information is lateralized in the right and left hemispheres respectively (see Chapter 1). The left hemiplegic patient (right side lesion) is more likely to have impaired visual memory, and the right hemiplegic (left side lesion) may show deficits in verbal memory. The assessment of visual and verbal memory is important in the development of appropriate strategies for adaptation of the patient's environment, and the choice of effective cues to be used by the therapist. Check-lists and daily planners, as well as cue cards for task sequencing, can be used in either pictorial or verbal form for verbal or visual deficits respectively. If there are problems in both modalities, audiotapes may be useful.

Assessment

Standardized

Doors and people (Baddeley et al., 1994)
Four subtests of long-term memory which can be used to separate visual and verbal memory.

(1) Visual recognition, using four photographs of doors.
(2) Visual recall based on patterns that are copied and later drawn from memory.
(3) Verbal recognition using names of people.
(4) Verbal recall based on the names of four people easily identified by profession.

Delayed recall is included to measure forgetting.

Computer assessment of memory
Computer software is available for the assessment of visual and verbal memory. The number of items in a display can be gradually increased, and either immediate or delayed recall can be tested (Fig. 13.1).

Functional
Activity analysis and task performance.

Compare performance in response to:

- written and verbal instructions
- visual instructions; line drawings or photographs.

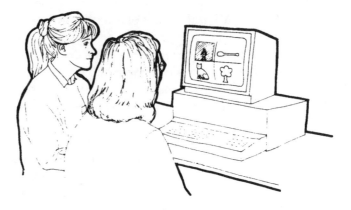

Fig. 13.1 Using computer assessment of memory.

Everyday memory

The assessment of memory in occupational therapy must be related to the patient's current environment and lifestyle. After cerebral damage some patients deny that they have a memory problem because their new environment makes few demands on memory. In the degenerative conditions of Alzheimer's and Korsakoff's diseases, the deterioration in memory may be gradual and difficult to separate from other cognitive changes.

Studies in neuropsychology have focused on the explanation of amnesia characterized by two main changes in long-term memory: loss of some memories acquired before onset, known as retrograde or premorbid amnesia; and difficulty in learning and remembering new information, known as anterograde or postmorbid amnesia.

Long-term memory loss is usually greatest for the time immediately preceeding the onset, and distant memories are often retained. Most recently, anterograde amnesia has been explained as a deficit in memory of the context of new information presented. The inability to learn names of people in the patient's postmorbid environment may be due to the loss of the contextual processing at the time of registration. This could account for the retained ability to retrieve premorbid memories of people and events, but it does not explain the temporal variations in retrograde memory loss.

The inability to learn new information makes the prospect for employment poor, especially when there is also a loss of semantic memory. Spared procedural memory retains the ability to perform skilled actions learnt in the past, although memory aids are needed for the parts of the activity that rely on semantic memory. The identification of a spared work or leisure skill may restore self-esteem and provide motivation for further memory training. Some patients may be able to learn new motor tasks, although they are often unaware of the changes (Parkin, 1996).

Daily living routine is affected by episodic and prospective memory loss. The patient cannot remember what he or she had for breakfast, or that a relative visited yesterday, because daily events cannot be coded in time and place (episodic). The inability to follow a TV programme which demands remembering what happened a few minutes before, or to recall a conversation with a friend, leads to social isolation from the family and friends. Omissions occur in the daily routine due to the loss of prospective memory which activates plans for action at the correct time. The person may fail to get dressed, or eat lunch or phone a member of the family.

Can everyday memory be standardized?

The Rivermead Behavioural Memory Test (RBMT) (Wilson *et al.*, 1991) was developed to provide an objective assessment of a range of everyday memory problems. The results of this battery of tests can be used to predict functional problems related to impairment of semantic, episodic and procedural memory covering verbal and visual memory. The tests have been standardized for the age range 16 to 64 years and for 65 to 96 years. The scores for the battery of tests allow for categorization into normal, poor memory, moderately impaired and severely impaired. Tests of semantic memory include recall of name, date, orientation, and recognition of pictures and faces. The ability to recall a short story, a route and a hidden belonging are tested, as well as prospective memory for an appointment. The effect of delayed recall can also be assessed by the repetition of some of the tests 20–25 minutes later.

Scores on the RBMT can be affected by an underlying perceptual problem, particularly remembering a route, and recognizing objects and faces. In a study of performance on the RBMT comparing patients with and without perceptual deficits (Cockburn *et al.*, 1990), no difference was found in the two groups in recognizing objects. This was probably due to the use of verbal memory in naming the objects, rather than visual memory. The authors, however, concluded that a shortened version of the RBMT should be used for patients who are unable to complete all the subtests due to perceptual deficits.

Table 13.1 Examples of the prediction of functional problems from memory tests.

Activity	Type of memory	Test
Orientation, time/place	Semantic	RBMT 10
Remember appointment	Prospective	RBMT 3, 4, 9
Follow TV programme	Working memory	Digit span
	Semantic, episodic	RBMT 6

Inspection of the scores in the individual tests of the RBMT can be used to predict where functional problems may occur. Conversely, the problem areas in functional activities for the individual patient can be listed. These activities can be related to the type of memory involved and then to the individual tests in the assessment battery. Examples are given in Table 13.1.

The functional assessment of memory loss requires observation of the patient over all times of the day, and in different settings if appropriate. Questionnaires have been used to provide information about the memory of an individual in relation to daily living. This method depends on the person's insight into his or her own cognitive abilities and ability to monitor his or her own performance. Questionnaires completed by the family, carer or members of the multi-disciplinary team may give more reliable information.

Assessment

Standardized

RBMT
There are 11 subtests, in four parallel versions for repeated testing, with norms for ages 16 to 96 years.
The subtests are: first name, second name, belonging, appointment, pictures, story (immediate and delayed), faces, route (immediate and delayed), message, orientation and date.

COTNAB, Section 4, III
Ability to follow spoken instructions.
A short spoken story is read to the patient, who is then asked to select 12 picture cards from a total of 25 cards to illustrate the story. The cards must be placed in the correct order (Fig. 13.2). Record:

- memory capacity from the amount of information that can be retained
- semantic and sequencing (episodic) errors.

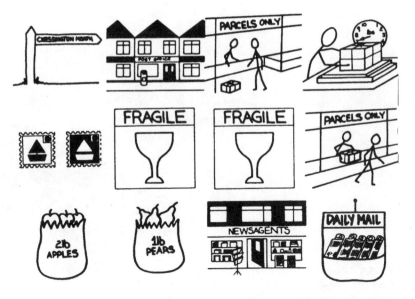

Fig. 13.2 Recall of a story in pictures – COTNAB Section 4 III. Reproduced in reduced size with permission of Nottingham Rehab.

Functional

- List functional activities that present problems due to memory loss. Identify the types of memory involved and relate to individual test scores in the RBMT.
- Prospective memory can be assessed by asking the patient to execute a previously agreed action, for example make a telephone call, at a specified time in the future. The interval between the request and the action can be gradually increased from minutes to hours or to the next day.

Compensation strategies

The outcome of memory assessment leads to the choice of compensation strategies which enable the memory-impaired person to function in their own environment. The application of internal strategies, for example mnemonics, paired associates and visual imagery, have limited application in daily living. Also, people with no memory impairment choose external strategies, for example diaries and wall planners, for prospective memory aids. The success of strategies devised to improve memory function depend on the awareness of the individual and on his or her cognitive ability to use memory aids.

Alarm watches and audiotapes can be used as prompts for the initiation and sequencing of tasks, respectively. Computerized memory aids may be successful for patients with premorbid experience of a

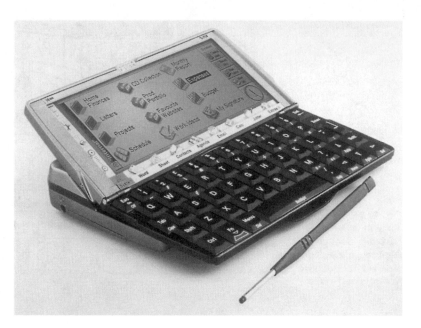

Fig. 13.3 Psion Organizer, Series 5. Photograph courtesy of Psion PLC.

personal computer. The Psion Organizer (Fig. 13.3) gives an alarm prompt and displays a message that gives the action required. A study by Wilson (1991) found that memory aids were being used by patients living independently five to ten years after traumatic brain injury. The author emphasized the need to teach memory aids in the environment in which they will be used.

The Contextual Memory Test (CMT) (Toglia, 1993) is a standardized assessment which is designed to measure both the awareness of memory capacity in task performance and the ability to use strategies to compensate for memory impairment. All the tests are related to function.

Assessment

Standardized

CMT

(1) Awareness of memory function. Questions are used to predict and estimate memory capacity before and after the observation of task performance respectively.
(2) Recall of line drawings of objects.
(3) Strategy use. Ability to use and benefit from an appropriate strategy.

Autobiographical memory

Autobiographical memory is a history which gives us our personal identity. The phrase 'we are what we remember' expresses clearly the importance of this aspect of everyday memory. People, places and objects are part of autobiographical memory as well as the events we have experienced. A vase on a shelf or a postcard in a drawer can vividly retrieve the memory of a holiday in the distant past with all the associated people and events. When this memory has gone, the sense of loss for the family and friends, as well as the person, is great.

Some autobiographical memories involve recall of declarative memory for a unique event, for example the facts about our first day at school. Specific memories of dramatic and emotional events have been called flashbulb memories. An example is hearing the news that Princess Diana had been killed in a car crash. Most people can remember when and where they were, and who told them. Flashbulb memories may have unique registration in memory, but the frequent rehearsal and retelling of the event may account for the accuracy of recall rather than a special mechanism. Other autobiographical memories may be more general, for example recall of schooldays from a schema or script developed over time which has been updated with experience of our own children at school.

Autobiographical memory has an important function in problem-solving activities. An example is my inability to remember the procedure for using jump leads in the car, but the recall of one evening when I left work to find the lights on and a flat battery acts as a cue for what I must do.

The orientation to person, place and social role is part of retrograde memory, and disorientation is sometimes associated with memory loss. The assessment of autobiographical memory can be useful in the planning of orientation and reminiscence for the memory-impaired patient.

The Autobiographical Memory Interview (AMI) (Kopelman et al., 1989) is a standardized assessment of personal remote memory, including its temporal gradient. Three periods of the patient's life are assessed in both parts: childhood; early adult life; and recent (in the last year). Some of the questions in the AMI may not be appropriate for the lifestyle or culture of the individual, but for a non-standardized test the format can be adapted by the therapist.

The assessment of autobiographical memory relies on consultation with relatives to provide information about important events in the patient's life span.

Assessment

Standardized

AMI
A semi-structured interview divided into two parts:

- Personal semantic schedule – recall of facts from the past.
- Autobiographical incidents schedule – recall of specific incidents in the patient's past.

Confabulation

Confabulation is a feature of memory impairment when the recall of autobiographical memory is apparently sensible, but untrue. Both the details and the context of a memory are confused, and the relationship of events in time is disrupted. Confabulation is not a simple loss of memories. Many dense amnesics do not confabulate, and those who do may show normal recall and recognition of semantic memory.

Retrieval of autobiographical memory involves the development of a strategy to activate stored knowledge with particular time and space dimensions. This is followed by a verification process as part of

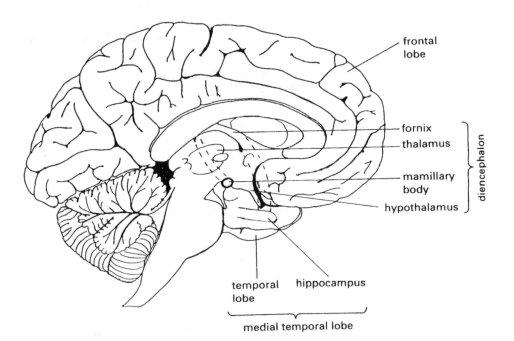

Fig. 13.4 Sagittal section of the brain to show the position of: the medial temporal lobe; the diencephalon; and the frontal lobe.

Table 13.2   Memory function related to brain areas.

Brain area	Type of memory	Cause of damage
Temporal lobe, hippocampus	Episodic memory, spatial memory (right)	Viral encephalitis, traumatic brain injury, CVA, anoxia
Diencephalon: thalamus, hypothalamus mamillary bodies	Procedural Autobiographical	Korsakoff's syndrome, cerebral tumours
Frontal lobes	Prospective memory Working memory Autobiographical memory	Traumatic brain injury, Korsakoff's syndrome, CVA, multiple sclerosis

retrieval which is analogous with problem-solving activity. Also, confabulation most frequently occurs in patients with frontal lobe lesions. The common features of processing and anatomical location suggest that confabulation may be a memory impairment with an overlay of dysexecutive syndrome (Chapter 15).

Summary of brain areas

The sagittal section of the brain (Fig. 13.4) passes through the slit-like third ventricle and the brain stem. The thalamus forms the wall of the third ventricle with the hypothalamus below. The medial border of the temporal lobe can be seen anterior to the brain stem.

The three main areas involved in memory are: the medial temporal lobes; the diencephalon; and the frontal lobes. Possible memory deficits have been related to each of these areas (Table 13.2).

References

Baddeley, A. D., Emslie, H. & Nimmo-Smith, I. (1994) *Doors and People*. Bury St Edmunds: Thames Valley Test Company.

Cockburn, J., Wilson, B. A., Baddeley, A. D. & Hiorns, R. (1990) Assessing everyday memory in patients with perceptual deficits. *Clinical Rehabilitation* **4**, 129–35.

Jonides, J., Smith, E. E., Koeppe, R. A., Awh, E., Minoshima, S. & Mintun, M. A. (1993) Spatial working memory in humans as revealed by PET. *Nature* **363**, 623–4.

Kopelman, M., Wilson, B. A. & Baddeley, A. D. (1989) The autobiographical memory interview: a new assessment of autobiographical and personal semantic memory in amnesic patients. *Journal of Clinical and Experimental Neuropsychology* **11**, 724–44.

Parkin, A. J. (1996) Chapter 9, Amnesia. In *Explorations in Cognitive Neuro-psychology*. Oxford: Blackwell Publishers.

Paulesu, E., Frith, C. D. & Frackowiak, R. S. J. (1993) The neural correlates of the verbal component of working memory. *Nature* **362**, 342–5.

Robinson, S. (1992) Occupational therapy in a memory clinic. *British Journal of Occupational Therapy* **55**, 394–6.

Toglia, J. P. (1993) *Contextual Memory Test*. San Antonio, TX: Therapy Skill Builders.

Wilson, B. A. (1991) Long-term prognosis of patients with severe memory disorders. *Neuropsychological Rehabilitation* **1**, 117–34.

Wilson, B. A., Cockburn, J. & Baddeley, A. D. (1991) *The Rivermead Behavioural Memory Test*. Bury St Edmunds: Thames Valley Test Company.

Further reading

Wilson, B. A. & Moffat, N. (eds) (1992) *Clinical Management of Memory Problems*. London: Chapman Hall.

Chapter 14 Dyspraxia

Apraxia is a disorder in the performance of meaningful learned movement. Most of the definitions in the literature are based on the exclusion of muscle weakness, incoordination, sensory loss or incomprehension, which could otherwise account for the problems observed in the execution of the movements.

The disorders named as apraxias include: buccofacial, constructional, dressing, gait, gaze, limb and speech apraxia. The term 'apraxia' is applied to each of these disorders, many of which are unrelated in their origin and presentation. Concha (1987) separates constructional apraxia as a spatial deficit with an added problem of planning and initiating movements. Dressing apraxia is now often interpreted as a spatial and body scheme disorder. Constructional and dressing apraxia were both considered in Chapter 11. Both buccofacial and limb apraxia present as the inability to make meaningful movements of the face or the limbs respectively. Nevertheless, there is reason to separate buccofacial from limb apraxia on the grounds of the contribution of the limbic system to the innervation of the facial muscles, whose movements are largely associated with the expression of emotion.

In neuropsychology, apraxia has been broadly defined as a disorder of the expressive functions (Lezak, 1983), namely speaking, manipulating, gesturing and facial expressions. The apraxias are then the deficits in the meaningful movements associated with the expressive functions.

In occupational therapy, patients are observed making purposeful movements, usually of the upper limbs, in task performance. When problems occur that cannot be explained by: the exclusion factors given above; or visual and spatial deficits, the term dyspraxia is used clinically. Some of these patients perform routine tasks in the home environment without difficulty, but problems may arise when they are asked to do apparently the same activity to command in a different environment. In addition, single movements to reach, to point, to grasp, to lift, and so on may be performed without errors, but disordered movement is seen when simple actions are combined into a sequence of actions to perform a task, especially when multiple objects are used.

In this chapter, the term limb dyspraxia will be used to describe the deficits in the movements associated with object use in the performance of daily living tasks. The origin of the dyspraxia will be considered in the framework of: the conceptual (semantic) knowledge object use and the actions related to them; linked to, the motor planning and execution of the appropriate movements (see Chapter 7).

Action errors in limb dyspraxia

In a review of studies of apraxia in neuropsychology over nearly a century, Tate & McDonald (1995) concluded that a definitive account of this syndrome remains an enigma. There was a lack of consistency in the features of the action errors described by different authors, and a wide range in the number of errors suggested as criteria for the diagnosis. These differences can only be resolved by a consensus of opinion on what constitutes an error, based on detailed analysis and recording of error types (York & Cermak, 1995).

Both quantitative and qualitative analysis of the errors have been used. A simple quantitative approach would use correct/incorrect records on a check-list of simple tasks using familiar objects in different conditions. This gives an overall indication of the severity of the problem but no information about where the movement breaks down. Qualitative measures require a clear description of both what constitutes an error and of the different types of errors that may be observed. The descriptions must also be valid across different patients, tasks and observers.

Alexander *et al.* (1992) identified six error types arranged hierarchically in order of increased disruption of movement: no movement, perseveration, undifferentiated movement, spatial error, body part as object, verbalization/self-cue. Schwartz *et al.* (1995) and Foundas *et al.* (1995) included sequencing errors, for example omissions, blending of elements and incorrect order. There is more agreement on the conditions in which dyspraxia should be observed. These include:

(1) Object-oriented movement, with the object present (transitive) and without the object (intransitive):
   • on verbal command (pantomime)
   • by imitation (copying the therapist)
   • using objects in a multi-step task.

(2) Symbolic gestures which are meaningful, e.g. wave goodbye; or meaningless, e.g. make a fist:
- on verbal command
- by imitation (copying the therapist).

The description of praxis based on two levels of processing (see Chapter 7) has led to the separation of dyspraxia into two types, i.e. ideational and ideomotor, originally defined by Liepmann. This continues to influence current research, and it has clinical significance for the diagnosis and treatment of dyspraxia. The features of the ideational and ideomotor types of dyspraxia will now be considered.

Ideational type

Ideational dyspraxia is defined as a disorder in the performance of purposeful movement due to a loss of the conceptual (semantic) knowledge of movement related to objects. The patient makes errors when using objects and tools in routine task performance or on command. Ideational dyspraxic patients may be able to name and to describe the function of objects, but cannot integrate this knowledge with the actions related to their use.

Single actions, such as putting a plug into a socket, or turning on a tap, may be done fluently and accurately in familiar surroundings. The situation changes when an activity involves sequencing and the use of more than one object (Fig. 14.1). Critical steps in the sequence may be omitted (e.g. stirring a coffee mug with no water in it); or two parts of the sequence may be blended together (e.g. pouring the coffee into the mug rather than spooning it).

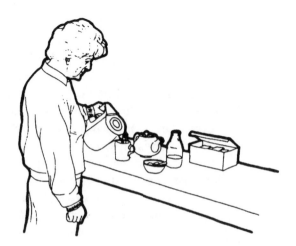

Fig. 14.1 Task using multiple objects.

Lehmkuhl & Poeck (1981) described the primary problem in ideational apraxia as the inability to perform the serial ordering of actions using multiple objects. A group of patients with ideational apraxia were asked to arrange photographs in the correct order to illustrate tasks requiring the use of several objects. This group performed significantly worse than a group of patients without ideational apraxia. When the photographs illustrated everyday events there was no difference between the two groups.

More recent studies distinguish ideational apraxia as an 'agnosia of usage' which is a loss of the knowledge of the use of objects (Ochipa et al., 1992). This results in a mismatch between object and action. A dyspraxic patient described by Miller (1986) attempted to pour himself a drink of orange squash by first pouring without unscrewing the top of the bottle, then continuing to pour with the cap removed, and finally emptying it into the water jug instead of the glass. In testing dyspraxic patients away from their normal surroundings, the ideational dyspraxic may perform a recognizable action, but inappropriate for the object presented. When given a pencil, the movements performed may be those for combing the hair.

Perseveration of an action may be seen in ideational apraxia, for example placing the teacup on a saucer and then repeating the action putting the teapot on a saucer. Overshooting a component of a task is seen in errors such as filling a glass with cordial instead of leaving space for the water. Some ideational dyspraxic patients are unaware of the errors they are making and are in danger of causing accidents, such as leaving gas unlit on the cooker by the omission of lighting the match. In other cases, the patient is aware of the errors being made, but can do nothing to correct them. They may be wrongly labelled as confused.

Ideomotor type

Ideomotor dyspraxia is defined as a disorder in the selection, timing, and spatial organization of purposeful movement. The ideomotor dyspraxic patient cannot carry out what is intended, even though the conceptual (semantic) knowledge of action is intact.

Errors are made when the patient is asked to perform object-oriented movements, both on verbal command and by imitation (copying) of the therapist. The spatial and temporal features of the movements are most affected.

When asked to demonstrate object use (without the object present), the patient may use a body part as the missing object, known as BPO. For example, in the actions for brushing the teeth, a finger may be used as a toothbrush and rubbed against the teeth (Fig. 14.2a). The plane of movement may be altered, e.g. shaving with the razor moving horizontally (Fig. 14.2b); or there may be poor distal differentiation of movement, e.g. the hand is held in a neutral position when performing gestures.

Perseveration of action may occur, particularly at transition points from one action to another in the sequence. For example, in lighting the cooker, perseveration of the action of striking the match may occur before turning on the gas tap. Gestural enhancement and vocal overflow are often observed during the demonstration of object use. Using a hammer, the body may rock backwards and forwards or there may be vocalization of 'bang, bang'.

Performance improves when the object is held in the hand. The additional sensory input from the object, and the constraints of movement imposed by it, both facilitate the execution of the movements (Concha, 1987).

In the familiar home environment, there may be no problems with routine tasks that can be completed automatically. When the attention demands increase, the movements lack fluency and look clumsy. This can often be a source of irritation and frustration to the patient and the family. In the absence of other problems, the patient can function reasonably well at home, but safety is at risk.

Table 14.1 is a summary of the error types in limb dyspraxia.

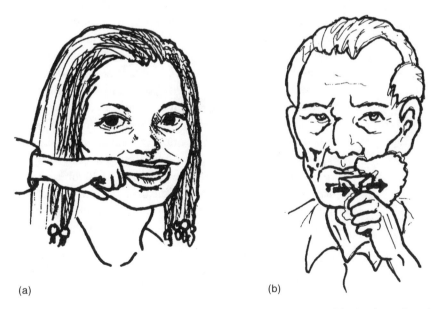

(a)   (b)

Fig. 14.2 Ideomotor dyspraxia: (a) cleaning teeth, body part as object; (b) shaving, altered proximity.

Table 14.1 Error types in ideational and ideomotor dyspraxia.

Ideational	Ideomotor
Poor performance on verbal command but can copy object-oriented movements	Poor performance to command and cannot copy object-oriented movements
Mismatch of object and action	Body part as object
Sequencing errors – wrong order, omissions, elements blended	Altered plane and proximity Poor distal differentiation
Overshoot, incomplete	Gestural enhancement Vocal overflow
Perseveration	Perseveration

Assessment with object or task?

Praxis problems are usually seen in left hemisphere lesion (right hemiplegia), but they can occur in lesion of either hemisphere (York & Cermak, 1995). The assessment of limb dyspraxia in a right hemiplegic patient may require him or her to perform the movements with the non-dominant hand. A former routine task now requires problem-solving ability and this needs to be borne in mind in the assessment.

Research studies of apraxia have assessed object-oriented movements either in a test situation or in a natural setting. In the development of a cognitive assessment, Bernspång et al. (1989) introduced a praxis test of object use in three conditions: to verbal command; by imitation; and in a bimanual multi-object task.

Schwartz et al. (1995) used five multi-step tasks, for example preparing toast and marmalade. Detailed analysis of the performances showed that the same patient may appear to be dyspraxic in one task and unimpaired in another, which emphasizes the need to assess across tasks and conditions. Foundas et al. (1995) videoed a group of dyspraxic patients over a period of 30 minutes during eating a meal placed on a lunch tray at the usual time and place. The authors recommend that dyspraxia should be assessed by observation of patients in natural settings, and that therapists should develop norms within their own clinical setting.

Both the severity and the functional implications of dyspraxia are most easily identified in the observation of the patient performing tasks. A qualitative assessment can be made in occupational therapy from the observation of a variety of relevant tasks, with familiar objects, on several different days.

Before the assessment of dyspraxia, abnormal tone, paresis, unilateral neglect and hemianopia should all be excluded. Early consultation with the speech and language therapist is important to screen for language deficits.

Assessment

Standardized

LOTCA
Praxis test B 8 (symbolic and object-oriented actions) motor imitation, utilization of objects, and symbolic actions. Scoring: 1, unable to produce any task; 2, only able to imitate movements; 3, able to imitate movements and to manipulate objects; 4, performs all tasks.

Functional

Matching of objects by function
In an appropriate setting, the patient is asked to choose two objects which have the same function. For example:
In the bathroom – which objects can be used to wash the face?
In the kitchen – which objects can be used to: (a) cut food into pieces; (b) pour water into a bowl?
Patients without language problems can be asked to describe the function of a presented object, or to draw an object that has a named use.

Object-oriented movement
Familiar objects are chosen and presented to the patient, one at a time, for example toothbrush, comb, scissors. The object-oriented movements are tested under three conditions:

(1)   On command, 'pretend to use this object' (object not held).
(2)   By imitation, 'copy the actions I use for this object'.
(3)   Object in the hand, 'demonstrate the use of this object'.

Ideational – poor object matching
            – can imitate actions, but not on command.
Ideomotor – normal matching by function
            – poor performance on command and imitation.

Task-oriented movement

Choose tasks ranging from simple to complex (multi-object). Observe the patient performing the tasks in a familiar setting, and in an unfamiliar setting if possible. Repeat on different days.

Identify whether the performance breaks down due to:

(1) organization and sequencing errors – ideational type; or
(2) spatial, temporal and limb postural errors – ideomotor type.

Record errors on a check-list (see Table 14.1).

Summary of brain areas

The following summary gives a guide to the brain areas associated with dyspraxia (Fig. 14.3).

- *Left parietal lobe* – ideational type.
- *Left frontal lobe* – ideomotor type (right hand).
- *Right frontal lobe* – ideomotor type (left hand).
- *Corpus callosum* – the same as for right frontal lobe.

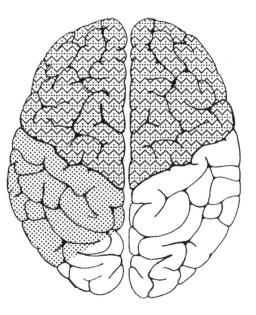

Fig. 14.3 Brain areas associated with dyspraxia of the ideational and ideomotor types.

References

Alexander, M. P., Baker, E., Naeser, M. A., Kaplan, E. & Palumbo, C. (1992) Neuropsychological and neuroanatomical dimensions of ideomotor apraxia. *Brain* **115**, 87–107.

Bernspång, B., Viitanen, M. & Eriksson, S. (1989) Impairments of perceptual and motor functions. Their influence on self-care ability 4–6 years after stroke. *Occupational Therapy Journal of Research* **9**, 27–37.

Concha, M. E. (1987) A review of apraxia. *British Journal of Occupational Therapy* **50**(7), 222–6.

Foundas, A. L., Macauley, B. L., Raymer, A. M., Maher, L. M., Heilman, K. M. & Rothi, L. J. G. (1995) Ecological implications of limb apraxia: evidence from mealtime behaviour. *Journal of the International Neuropsychological Society* **1**, 62–6.

Lehmkuhl, G. & Poeck, K. (1981) Conceptual organization and ideational apraxia. *Cortex* **17**, 153–8.

Lezak, M. D. (1983) *Neuropsychological Assessment*. New York: Oxford University Press.

Miller, N. (1986) *Dyspraxia and its Management*. London: Croom Helm.

Ochipa, C., Rothi, L. J. G. & Heilman, K. M. (1992) Conceptual apraxia in Alzheimer's disease. *Brain* **115**, 1061–71.

Schwartz, M. F., Fitzpatrick-DeSalme, E. J. & Carew, T. G. (1995) The Multiple Objects Test for ideational apraxia: aetiology and task effects on error profiles. *Journal of the International Neuropsychological Society* **1**, 149.

Tate, R. L. & McDonald, S. (1995) What is apraxia? The clinician's dilemma. *Neuropsychological Rehabilitation* **5**(4), 273–97.

York, C. D. & Cermak, S. A. (1995) Visual perception and praxis in adults after stroke. *American Journal of Occupational Therapy* **49**(6), 543–50.

Further reading

Rothi, L. J. G. & Heilman, K. M. (eds) (1997) *Apraxia: The Neuropsychology of Action*. Hove: Psychology Press.

Chapter 15　Dysexecutive Syndrome

The executive functions of the brain are crucial to the planning and performance of action and behaviour that is not habitual for the particular individual. A large part of our daily living activity is routine and automatic. New skills that we have learnt as a result of practice, for example driving, typing and speaking a second language, are also automatic. When we are confronted by a new situation or an unfamiliar task, executive processing is involved in setting a goal, planning and organizing action and behaviour.

Dysexecutive syndrome (DES) (formerly known as frontal lobe syndrome) is the result of deficits in the executive system which directs and regulates all the other cognitive systems. There are many different features of dysexecutive syndrome so that it is identified by a cluster of symptoms rather than a clearly defined syndrome. The patient with DES may present as apathetic, inflexible and unable to initiate any activity without instructions. On the other hand, he or she may show impulsivity, distractibility and loss of control of ongoing behaviour.

The prefrontal cortex has been identified as the localization of executive processing based on PET scan studies of normal subjects and the observation of the behaviour of patients with frontal lobe lesions. However, the anatomical links of the frontal lobes with other regions of the cerebral cortex and with subcortical brain areas means that executive functions cannot be solely localized in one brain area.

The patient with DES has difficulty in grasping the whole of a complicated state of affairs. He or she may be able to work along routine lines, but cannot master new situations. In task performance, some of the features of DES are similar to dyspraxia. However, while ideomotor dyspraxic patients can usually function automatically in a familiar environment, patients with DES may not be able to organize themselves to start any activity. Many patients with DES also have memory and attention problems. Pure amnesics without DES can still organize themselves by using memory aids; those with DES cannot.

Action and behaviour in dysexecutive syndrome

Dysexecutive syndrome is commonly seen after traumatic brain injury. Individual patients present with a variety of behavioural changes. Loss of affect, lack of motivation, inappropriate social behaviour and lack of insight are all factors which may compound the overall disorganization of behaviour. The cognitive effects of DES will be considered. The reader is asked to look elsewhere for information on psychosocial issues. Task performance requires self-initiation, at a different level of control from initiation in the motor system (Chapter 7). Starting to eat food on a plate is different from preparing food when hungry which requires planning ability. Effective planning includes a strategy or routine that can be activated when conditions change, and the ability to maintain it until the goal is reached.

The estimation of task difficulty and the knowledge of time to complete the task is also part of planning. Impulsivity is seen in some patients with DES who cannot plan and maintain what they intended to do.

Once activity is initiated, perseveration may occur when contention scheduling is strongly triggered by the environment and the response persists in the absence of control by the executive system. Alternatively, the patient may be 'stimulus bound' and unable to change to a different response if the conditions alter. The Wisconsin Card Sorting Test (Milner, 1963) is designed to assess this executive function. The patient is asked to sort cards that have stimuli which vary by shape and colour (Fig. 15.1).

At first, the subject sorts the cards by one particular rule, for example red crosses. After six successful applications, the rule is

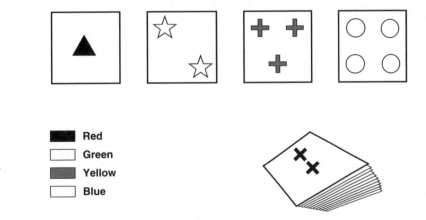

Fig. 15.1 Wisconsin Card Sorting Test, showing the material as presented to the subject. Reproduced with permission from Milner, B. (1963) *Archives of Neurology* **9**, 90–100. Copyright 1963, American Medical Association.

changed to a different stimulus, for example green stars. The DES patient continues to sort by the first rule even when told it is wrong. In daily living this presents as an inability to respond to changing situations, or to shift from one task to another.

Underlying attention deficits are often a feature of DES (see the sections entitled 'Sustained attention', 'Selective attention' and 'Divided attention' in Chapter 5). Loss of orientation to time of day, seasons and situations is an indication of poor alertness to environmental cues. When attention is captured, the DES patient may become stimulus bound and cannot manipulate or direct his or her gaze to more than one thing at a time. Distractibility is seen when there are no strong triggers in the environment to activate contention scheduling and responses are made to irrelevant stimuli.

Poor functional performance can neither be recognized nor corrected if there is loss of self-awareness and self-reflectiveness. These problems relate to the metacognition level in the model by Sohlberg *et al.* (1993) (see Chapter 8) which includes knowing how to attend, to organize and to solve problems. When asked to write a description of a familiar activity, a patient with DES may produce a list of unrelated features.

Functional problems experienced in DES may be less obvious when the patient is in hospital or in a rehabilitation centre, where there is structure to the day, and there is little need to use initiative or to take responsibility. The situation changes when the patient is discharged to a home environment where this structure is absent and support from the family, carer or community occupational therapist becomes essential.

Functional assessment of dysexecutive syndrome

The component skills of the executive system have been listed under headings by different authors in the literature (Ben-Yishay & Diller, 1983; Lezack, 1983; Ylvisaker & Szekeres, 1989; Zoltan, 1996). These lists of executive skills can be used as a basis for structured observation in a functional assessment of dysexecutive syndrome. Some of the component areas may be intact while problems are observed in other areas. The outcome of the assessment is a profile of the executive functions for the individual client which can be used as a basis for treatment planning.

A check-list of components is used by the therapist during observation of a patient performing a multi-step task, which is non-routine but relevant to the patient's current lifestyle. Information about the client's premorbid lifestyle obtained from family and friends is an important part of functional assessment. This task analysis approach identifies where breakdown occurs in the activity. The profile can be used to predict how the patient will perform in daily living, leisure and work activities.

The choice of task for the functional assessment must be at the appropriate level of difficulty and one that the client is likely to be able to complete. At a severe level of DES the task may be washing, dressing or organizing breakfast. At an intermediate level the task may be making a two-course meal including the shopping and the budgeting. A high-level individual may plan an outing for a group, or plan and give a presentation on a familiar topic. Construction tasks, for example making a wooden toy, offer a good opportunity to observe the components of executive function. A check-list approach can be used to record how the client plans the task and the way he or she deals with problems during the execution. Information about planning, organizing, impulsivity and rigidity can be noted. Some clients may use the same problem-solving approach over and over again, even if it is wrong.

The eight components described by Ylvisaker & Szekeres (1989) will now be considered and then used to compose the functional assessment.

(1)   Realistic goal-setting depends on the awareness of the client's own strengths and weaknesses and the estimation of task difficulty. This may be done by asking the client to rate how well he or she thinks the task will be done on a scale of 1 to 10.

(2)   Planning is the ability to plan the steps involved to reach the goal. The steps must be executed in the correct sequence to reach the goal. Planning problems lead to impulsive and rigid behaviour with poor time sense.

(3)   Organizing is related to carrying out the plan. Knowledge of the strategies that may be needed if conditions change is part of organizing. The appreciation of situations when assistance is required may be part of the planning.

(4)   Self-initiating is the ability to spontaneously start the task. The level achieved depends on the amount of structure and cueing required for initiation by the client. A task may be set to complete in the client's own time before the next OT session.

(5)   Self-directing is needed to continue with the task once it has been initiated without seeking reassurance or direction from other people.

(6)   Self-correcting/self-monitoring. Self-correction is the ability to put something right that has gone wrong. The anticipation of errors requires self-monitoring, so that the course of action is altered to avoid something going wrong. The DES patient may have difficulty in learning from mistakes.

(7)   Flexible problem-solving involves the processing of all the relevant information, and decision-making about the most effective solution. Problem-solving includes the ability to think of more than one solution to a problem. The DES patient who has learnt new skills cannot transfer them to new situations.

(8)   Self-inhibiting is the basis of turn-taking in action and behaviour. Verbal and non-verbal behaviour requires self-inhibiting for listening, and for responding at the appropriate time and place. This can be assessed in a group situation and in cooperation with the speech and language specialist.

Assessment

Functional

Choose a non-routine multi-step activity, at a level that can be completed and is familiar to the client.

The following check-list of the component executive skills is structured with suggested questions to form a basis for therapist/client discussion before the start. Therapist observation occurs during the task, and feedback at the end.

Component executive skill	Questions
(1) Realistic goal-setting	What do you intend to do? Do you think you can do it now? How long will it take?
(2) Planning	Take me through all the steps in doing the activity? Are there any alternative steps?
(3) Organizing	Do you have the equipment you need? Do you need help from another person?
(4) Self-initiating	When will you begin the task? Shall I tell you when to start?
(5) Self-directing	Shall I give you prompts during the task? Shall I tell you when the task is going well?

(6) Self-correcting/   What problem may you
      self-monitoring   encounter?
                                  How would you overcome it?

(7) Flexible problem-solving   Can this activity be done in
                                    more than one way?

At the end: Have you achieved your goal
                                    for the activity?

Standardized

Behavioural Assessment of Dysexecutive Syndrome (BADS)
(Wilson et al., 1996)
A standardized test battery of six tests:

(1) Temporal judgement – estimate how long events last.
(2) Rule shift cards – ability to change response pattern.
(3) Action programme – practical problem-solving.
(4) Key search – strategy formation.
(5) Zoo map – route planning.
(6) Six elements test – schedule time to work on six tasks.

The battery also includes a Dysexecutive Questionnaire, one for
the patient and one for the carer. There are 20 items including
emotional, motivational, behavioural and cognitive changes
which are rated on a five-point scale.

COTNAB Section 4 (ability to follow instructions)
I   Make a coat hanger on a standard jig (written instruction).
II   Construct a metal assembly (visual instructions).

Cognitive Assessment of Minnesota (CAM) – cognitive screening
Five sections assess moderate to severe DES:
6 – temporal awareness; 14 – foresight and planning; 15 – safety
and judgement; 16 – concrete problem-solving; 17 – abstract
reasoning.

Summary of brain areas

The brain areas associated with the executive functions are the
prefrontal cortex and the cingulate cortex in the frontal lobes
(Fig. 15.2). The prefrontal cortex lies anterior to the primary motor
and pre-motor areas. It has reciprocal feedback connections with: the
primary motor and pre-motor areas; sensory areas of the parietal,
temporal and occipital lobes; and with the limbic system.

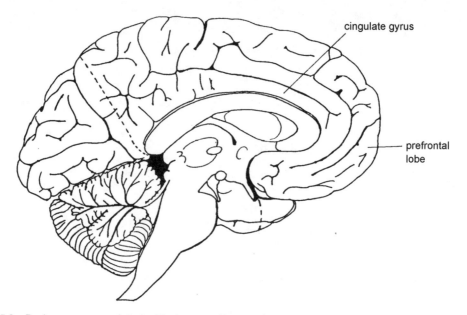

Fig. 15.2   Brain areas associated with dysexecutive syndrome.

References

Ben-Yishay, Y. & Diller, L. (1983) Cognitive remediation. In *Rehabilitation of the Head-Injured Adult* (E. Griffin, M. Bond & J. Miller, eds). Philadelphia: F. A. Davis.

Lezak, M. D. (1983) *Neuropsychological Assessment*. New York: Oxford University Press.

Milner, B. (1963) Effects of different brain lesions on card sorting. *Archives of Neurology* **9**, 90–100.

Sohlberg, M. M., Mateer, C. & Stuss, D. T. (1993) Contemporary approaches to the management of executive control dysfunction. *Journal of Head Trauma Rehabilitation* **8**(1), 45–58.

Wilson, B. A., Alderman, N., Burgess, P., Emslie, H. & Evans, J. J. (1996) *Behavioural Assessment of the Dysexecutive Syndrome (BADS)*. Bury St Edmunds: Thames Valley Test Company.

Ylvisaker, M. & Szekeres, S. F. (1989) Metacognitive and executive impairments in head-injured children and adults. *Topics in Language Disorders* **9**(2), 34–49.

Zoltan, B. (1996) *Vision, Perception and Cognition*. New Jersey: Slack Inc.

Appendix 1 Index of Standardized Assessments

Appendix 2 Summary of the Possible Cognitive Deficits Associated with Cerebral Lesion Sites

Note: Multiple lesion sites occur in many neurological conditions, and the outcome of lesion in one area varies widely in different individuals.

Site	Dominant (left)	Non-dominant (right)
Frontal lobe	dysexecutive syndrome limb dys/apraxia (ideomotor) verbal memory deficit – (working, prospective)	dysexecutive syndrome limb dys/apraxia (ideomotor) visual memory deficit – (working, prospective) premotor unilateral neglect sustained attention deficit
Parietal lobe	visual object agnosia – (associative) constructional apraxia body scheme disorder – (somatognosia) limb dys/apraxia (ideational)	visual object agnosia – (apperceptive) constructional deficits body scheme disorder – (anosognosia) topographical disorientation unilateral visual neglect selective attention deficit
Occipital lobe	right hemianopia visual perceptual deficits object agnosia, prosopagnosia – (bilateral)	left hemianopia visual perceptual deficits
Temporal lobe	prosopagnosia topographical disorientation memory deficit (episodic)	prosopagnosia topographical disorientation memory deficit (spatial and episodic)

Glossary

The prefixes 'a' and 'dys' are used interchangeably in describing deficits. Their literal meanings are 'inability to' and 'impairment of', respectively.

achromatopsia   inability to recognize colour, in the absence of retinal defects.

affordance   possibility for action provided by a surface or an object.

agnosia   inability to recognize familiar objects, in the absence of sensory impairment.

   apperceptive   failure to recognize familiar objects as a result of visual perceptual impairment.

   associative (semantic)   inability to integrate object percept with knowledge of object meaning and function.

agraphia   inability to produce meaningful written words.

alertness   an endogenous 'prepared for action' state which results in faster response time to stimuli.

alexia   reading disorder.

allocentric   spatial representations of the environment, irrespective of body position.

amnesia   partial or complete loss of memory.

   amnesic syndrome   global deterioration in memory function due to non-degenerative brain lesion.

   anterograde   difficulty in remembering new information acquired after brain damage.

   retrograde   loss of memory for a variable period of time prior to the onset of brain damage.

anomia   inability to name objects and faces.

anosognosia   inability to recognize a part of one's own body.

aphasia   inability to process spoken language.

apraxia (dyspraxia)   inability to make purposeful movements (in the presence of normal sensation and muscle tone).

   ideational   loss of the concept of movement (i.e. semantic knowledge related to action).

   ideomotor   disorder in the timing and spatial organization of purposeful movement.

arousal   physiological level of attention based on the activity in the reticular formation of the brain stem.

articulatory loop   subvocal rehearsal of speech-based information in working memory.

astereognosis (tactile agnosia)   inability to recognize objects from touch without vision.

attention   active processing directed to particular sensory stimuli for perceptual analysis.

divided   ability to switch attention between the stimuli associated with two different tasks.

selective   orienting to the relevant sensory stimuli (visual or auditory) in the environment.

sustained   endogenous attention maintained over a period of time (includes arousal and alertness).

autobiographical memory   long-term memory that is unique to the individual.

ballistic movement (*see* **open loop**)   action that is preprogrammed and cannot be modified once it has begun.

body image   subjective perception of the appearance of one's own body.

body scheme   perception of the relative position of the body parts.

bottom-up assessment   the focus on the impairment of components of the cognitive system which affect occupational performance.

bottom-up processing   begins with the perceptual analysis of sensory inputs and builds upwards towards the final stage of interpretation.

CAT scan   computerized axial tomography. A thin fan-shaped X-ray beam views a 'slice' of the brain. The X-ray tube revolves round the patient so that the brain is viewed from all angles. A computer combines all the views, and the changes in soft tissue at the lesion site are revealed in a single image.

central executive   control system that allocates attention between the visuospatial and phonological components of working memory.

cerebrovascular accident (event), (CVA)   a rapidly developing focal lesion in the brain that is vascular in origin.

closed loop   action that is modified during progress in response to internal and external feedback.

'cocktail party phenomenon'   the way we attend to some stimuli and ignore others.

coding   mental processing of information during learning.

cognitive system   a set of mental operations performed to reach a common goal.

colour constancy   tendency for a colour to look the same under a wide variation of lighting and viewing conditions.

concept   the stored mental representations of a set of objects, actions or events that share certain characteristics.

confabulation   recall of episodic or autobiographical memory that is apparently sensible but untrue.

constructional apraxia   difficulty in the organization of complex actions in two- or three-dimensional space.

contention scheduling   mechanism for the activation of a stored schema, triggered by the environment, with inhibition of competing schemas.

context   the particular circumstances in which an event or action takes place.

declarative memory   long-term memory for facts, incidents and events, that are retrieved by conscious access.

dissociation   the separation of one module of processing that is impaired when others are spared.

double dissociation   two modules of processing which can be selectively impaired.

dressing apraxia   inability to dress oneself, primarily due to a disorder of spatial perception and/or body scheme.

dysexecutive syndrome   impairment of the executive functions of the brain which is associated with frontal lobe lesion.

egocentric   spatial representations of the environment with regard to the position of the head and body.

episodic memory   long-term memories linked to a time and place.

everyday memory   memory function related to daily living.

executive functions   the mental operations involved in: goal-setting; organizing, monitoring and completing; action and behaviour.
   central executive   a component of working memory.

explicit memory   memory processes with awareness, assessed by tests of direct recall and recognition.

figure ground   the isolation of a shape or an object from its background.

form constancy   the perception of a familiar shape or object as the same, regardless of its position or the distance from which it is viewed.

gestalt   unified whole that is not revealed by simply analysing the parts.

hemianopia   'blindness' in part of the visual field of one or both eyes, originating in the pathway from the retina to the occipital cortex. *homonymous hemianopia*   'blindness' in the right or left side visual fields of both eyes.

hemiplegia   weakness or spasticity in the muscles of one side of the body, resulting from a lesion in the opposite side of the brain.

hippocampus   a buried gyrus in the temporal lobe of the brain involved in memory and spatial orientation.

implicit memory   memory that is not directly revealed in tests of recall and recognition.

lesion (brain)   change in the tissue of the brain resulting from vascular accident, trauma, disease or degeneration.

lexicon   store of known words.

long-term memory   memory that stores and processes information over periods of time from a few minutes to many years.

memory trace   neurological processing for a relatively permanent memory.

modality   a sensory system, e.g. visual modality, tactile modality.

module   a stage in the information processing of one particular perceptual or cognitive ability, for example object recognition.

MRI   magnetic resonance imaging. A strong magnetic field is produced by electromagnets distributed around the head. A radio pulse excites the hydrogen atoms in the water in the brain tissue. A computer translates the signals from the movement of the hydrogen atoms into an image, which identifies where lesions have occurred.

myelin   fatty sheath around axons of neurones in the white matter of the central nervous system, and in peripheral nerves, which increases the rate of conduction of nerve impulses.

neglect syndrome   failure to orient, report or respond to stimuli on one side of space (contralateral to the side of brain lesion).

neuro-imaging   scanning techniques which show the structure and/or the rate of local blood flow in brain areas; see CAT, MRI and PET scanning.

object-centred description   representation of the visual structure of an object, irrespective of viewpoint.

object constancy   the tendency for objects to be perceived as the same, even though they are observed in a variety of conditions, e.g. distance, orientation, location or lighting.

object-recognition units stored visual descriptions of all known objects.

open loop movement that cannot be modified once it has started, e.g. tap a key on a computer keyboard, throw a ball.

optic aphasia inability to name objects when presented visually, but can name from a verbal description and can gesture the use of the object.

paradigm a particular experimental procedure that is described in detail.

perseveration tendency to continue a particular action, word or pattern of behaviour, when the stimulus has been removed.

phonological store temporary storage of speech-based information in working memory.

positron emission tomography, PET scan reveals the level of activity in the different areas of the brain over time. A solution containing a radioactive isotope is injected intravenously and accumulates in the brain in amounts proportional to the local blood flow. The positrons emitted by the isotope are detected by sensors placed around the head.

praxis means, literally, movement. In neuropsychology the term applies to meaningful actions and gestures.

prefrontal cortex area of the frontal lobe anterior to the motor areas, associated with the executive functions.

procedural memory long-term memory for mental and motor skills that are retrieved without conscious awareness.

prosopagnosia inability to recognize familiar faces, in the presence of intact visual perception and object recognition.

prospective memory memory for future actions without obvious external cues.

representation neural activity in the processing of a member of a conceptual category.

stored memory as it has been in the past.

structural as it is now.

saccade a fast eye movement between two fixation points occurring in scanning and reading.

scanning the exploration of space by eye movements.

schema a packet of stored knowledge related to the same situation, which may incorporate actions, events or behaviours. Schemas act as plans for future behaviours.

semantic related to meaning.

semantic memory long-term memory for general knowledge and facts.

somatognosia failure to perceive how the body parts relate to each other, and their relative positions in space (disorder of body scheme).

spatial relations syndrome a severe spatial deficit in all aspects of spatial perception.

structural description specification of the parts of an object and the way they fit together; a framework for object recognition.

sulcus a fold in the surface of the brain.

central separates the frontal and parietal lobes.

lateral separates the temporal lobe from the frontal and parietal lobes.

supervisory attention system system for controlled attention in novel situations, or when decision-making is required.

syndrome a collection of symptoms that commonly occur together.

top-down assessment the focus on occupational roles and performance as a basis for compensation and adaptation in occupational therapy intervention.

top-down processing sequence of processes for the interpretation of information from the senses that are influenced by stored knowledge from past experience.

topographical disorientation inability to recall the spatial arrangement of familiar surroundings.

topographical memory memory for the landmarks and layout of familiar surroundings.

unilateral visual neglect inability to orient to visual stimuli in one side of space.

viewer-centred representation visual representation of an object from the viewpoint of the observer.

visual field area of the visual world that is visible out of the eye.

visuospatial sketchpad processing of visuospatial information in working memory.

working memory temporary storage of visuospatial and speech-based information controlled by an attentional system (central executive).

Index

verbal memory 129
  rehearsal 57
viral encephalitis 137
visual field 34–5
  defects 107–8, 122–4
visual memory 129
visual perception, basic 24–7, 98–100
  assessment 100–101
  colour 24–5, 99
  depth 25, 101

figure ground 25–6, 100
form 26–7, 100
visuospatial sketch pad, *see* working memory

Wernicke's area 4-5
working memory 56–8
  central executive 17, 57
  deficits 127–9
  phonological loop 57, 128
  visuospatial sketch pad 58, 128